Evaluating Mental-Health Programs: The Progress Evaluation Scales

Evaluating Mental-Health Programs: The Progress Evaluation Scales

David Ihilevich
Shiawassee County Community
Mental Health Center

Goldine C. Gleser
University of Cincinnati,
College of Medicine

LexingtonBooks
D.C. Heath and Company
Lexington, Massachusetts
Toronto

To Lenore J. Kroman

Library of Congress Cataloging in Publication Data

Ihilevich, David.
  Evaluating mental-health programs.

  Bibliography: p.
  Includes index.
  1. Mental health services—Evaluation. I. Gleser, Goldine C.
II. Title. III. Title: Progress evaluation scales. [DNLM:
1. Community mental health services—Organ. 2. Evaluation
studies—Methods. WM 30 I24e]
RA790.5.I38   616.89′14′0287   81–48627
ISBN 0–669–05464–x   AACR2

Published simultaneously in Canada

Printed in the United States of America

International Standard Book Number: 0–669–05464–x

Library of Congress Catalog Card Number: 81–48627

Project Personnel

David Ihilevich, Ph.D.
Project Director

Lenore J. Kroman, A.C.S.W.
Principal Investigator
University of Michigan
School of Social Work

Gordon W. Gritter, M.D.
Principal Investigator
Department of Psychiatry
Michigan State University

Goldine C. Gleser, Ph.D.
Project Consultant
Department of Psychiatry
University of Cincinnati

Andrew S. Watson, M.D.
Project Consultant
Department of Psychiatry and
   Law School
University of Michigan

Other Contributors

Robert R. Colyar, A.C.S.W.
Chief Psychiatric Social Worker
Shiawassee County CMH Center

Ronald N. Leuhrig, Ph.D.
Forensic Program Coordinator
Shiawassee County CMH Center

Keith Lyon, Ph.D.
Children & Adolescent Program
   Coordinator
Shiawassee County CMH Center

Robert M. Patterson, M.D.
Chief Psychiatrist
Shiawassee County CMH Center

Mary Louise Stimson, A.C.S.W.
Aftercare Program Coordinator
Shiawassee County CMH Center

Carol F. Rodvien, Ph.D.
Substance Abuse Program
   Coordinator
Shiawassee County CMH Center

Thomas West, A.C.S.W.
Forensic Program
Shiawassee County CMH Center

Kent C. Stoddard, A.C.S.W.
Developmental Disabilities
   Program Coordinator
Shiawassee County CMH Center

Phyllis Cooley, B.S.
Case Manager
Shiawassee County CMH Center

Alta M. Zahn, R.N.
Life Consultation Worker
Shiawassee County CMH Center

Contents

Figures

Tables

Preface

This book describes the development and standardization of a new evaluation system entitled the Progress Evaluation Scales (PES). This approach to evaluation was developed in order to overcome some of the major problems noted in other evaluation systems. The PES is made up of seven scales, each consisting of five levels, with the characteristics of each level described. Four slightly different versions of the scales are available to accommodate children, adolescent, and adult mental-health clients and, additionally, the developmentally disabled. The seven scales of the PES tap the areas of *Family Interaction, Occupation* (school-job-homemaking), *Getting Along with Others, Feelings and Mood, Use of Free Time, Problems,* and *Attitude toward Self.* The scales can be used to indicate both current-status functioning and goals and can be filled out by patient, therapist, and significant other. For the purpose of data analysis the five levels of each scale are assigned the numerical value of 1 to 5, from the most pathological to the healthiest levels of functioning observed in the community.

Results of extensive studies over an eight-year period indicate that the PES provides a fast and efficient measuring device for assessment of current status and change over time in clinically relevant aspects of personal, social, and community adjustment. The chief attributes of the scales follow.

1. Interviewers experienced in using the PES form can complete the scales in one to two minutes following a routine diagnostic interview. This factor is of considerable importance in gaining the cooperation of community mental-health-center staff both for adopting the scales for use on a continuous basis and for maintaining high quality of data gathered.

2. New staff from various professional disciplines joining a mental-health agency can easily learn how to use the scales and integrate them into their routine work with clients.

3. The one-page format, the colloquial language of the scales, and the simple procedures of administration make it possible for most community mental-health clients and their significant others to fill out the scales within five to eight minutes.

4. Comparisons of clients' ratings to those of their therapists and significant others, as well as comparisons of clients' own ratings over time, yield important ongoing information on the feelings, attitudes, and expectations of the principal people who affect the outcome of the therapeutic endeavor.

5. Generalizability of PES ratings with respect to raters and occasions has been examined for all four versions of the scales. Rater agreement

and stability over occasions have been found adequate for use in group comparisons. The average ratings of two separate interviewers are recommended for individual comparisons.

6. Construct validity studies reveal that the scales differentiate between normal and patient groups; differentiate among groups of various degrees of psychopathology; are by-and-large independent of demographic variables; relate, in the expected direction, to psychological constructs measured by other established inventories; meet criteria for convergent and discriminant validity on the basis of correlations between independent ratings of client or significant other and therapist; measure different domains of behavior and experience as indicated by the low intercorrelations among them; and are sensitive to changes in level of personal, social, and community adjustment as indicated by the independent ratings of therapists, patients, and significant others at the beginning, reevaluation, and termination of therapy.

7. Finally, the PES scales have extensive heuristic value for exploring important questions in the clinical, programmatic, and administrative and policy domains.

Acknowledgments

Foremost we wish to express our deep appreciation to all the members of the Shiawassee County Community Mental Health Services board for providing us with a balanced mixture of patience, support, and friendly, unintrusive encouragement. Without this evidence of trust and faith in us, this project could not have been carried out.

Dr. Gleser's research staff in Cincinnati should receive particular plaudits. They helped analyze data, typed progress reports, and put together the preliminary manuscript. In particular, our thanks go to Mary Danzeisen who typed the tables for this book and also typed the preliminary version of the manuscript. We also acknowledge our gratitude to Linda Crespo da Silva, Mary Grace, and Mary Kapp for their help in processing data.

The Shiawassee County Community Mental Health Center's secretarial staff deserves special acknowledgment. They helped us collect normative data, checked and rechecked in order to ensure that the scales were accurately transcribed, and promptly retyped endless "visions and revisions" of different sections of this manuscript. All this work was done above and beyond their regular duties. Their dedication, cohesiveness, and exemplary goodwill were both a challenge and an inspiration to us all. Thanks are due to Gertrude Cramner, Susan Blight, Nancy Durepo, Joan Durling, Sharon Fredrick, Gloria Gulick, Gayle Harris, Theodora Jacobs, Janet Lloyd, Joanne Rohde, and Elsie Yanik.

Thanks are also due to the many clients who contributed to the development of this project. Not only did they provide us with the raw material necessary to analyze the psychometric properties of the scales, but in addition, many of them reviewed preliminary drafts of the Progress Evaluation Scales and offered numerous valuable suggestions for the improvement of specific items.

We wish to acknowledge the financial assistance rendered us through a 314(d) federal grant and from the Michigan Department of Mental Health. Particularly impressive was the lack of any interference with our planning and execution of the project, the absence of red tape, artificial deadlines, and the like. Consequently, whatever we have achieved or failed to achieve in this project is due solely to our own abilities and limitations.

Finally, gratitude is due to the professional staff of the Shiawassee County Community Mental Health Center. This unique group of professionals shouldered the burden of planning, revising, and executing all phases of the project over eight years. But for their grace and unequivocal cooperation, the successful completion of this project would have been impossible. We are deeply appreciative of and grateful to each one of them.

1 Introduction

Review of Evaluation Methodologies

With the advent of deinstitutionalization over the past two decades and the massive shift of care to local communities, a growing clamor has developed for satisfactory methods to evaluate the quality of programs and services rendered at the community level. In the community mental-health field such demands for accountability culminated in the passage by Congress of Public Law 94-63, Community Mental Health Amendments of 1975, directing that 2 percent of the budget of all federally funded community mental-health centers be allocated for evaluation purposes.

Many mental-health professionals react defensively to such demands for accountability, countering that they are really a reflection of society's deep-seated ambivalence toward treating the mentally ill in the community or that such demands constitute shrewdly disguised rationalizations for cutting funds from vulnerable public programs that lack vocal, organized constituencies. Actually, mental-health professionals feel caught in the dilemma of responding to demands for accountability in the face of a body of literature yielding conflicting scientific evidence for the value of their psychotherapeutic services in significantly influencing clients' behavior in the direction therapists intend. This conflicting evidence is well summarized in a review of outcome studies of psychotherapy by Bergin and Suinn (1975), as well as in an analysis of evaluation studies that concluded, "program evaluation is still clearly in its infancy as a field of study" (Perloff, Perloff, and Sussna 1976: 156).

Four major difficulties have been encountered in providing scientific evidence for the value of therapeutic interventions. First, ethical contraints for experimentation with human beings do not allow for the scientific manipulation of various conditions, such as family relationships, dating behavior, friendships, or personal income, all of which probably have an important influence on the outcome of psychotherapy. Second, meaningful matching of patients for specific combinations of inherited endowment, past experience, and current environment is beyond the scope of any available technology. Third, there has been a lack of uniformity in the implied or explicit goals of different psychotherapeutic techniques and in the methods used to measure outcomes. And finally, standardized instruments for measuring outcome that are reliable, valid, and relevant

1

for clinical and programmatic decision making yet are sufficiently broad to be applicable to the great variety of programs and clients served by mental-health professionals in the community are largely unavailable.

Since the first two constraints are likely to be permanent conditions, outcome studies will probably never be definitive. The optimal conditions one can establish for such studies entail matching of subjects on a few variables believed to be relevant to therapy outcome (such as diagnosis, education, or motivation for change), random assignment of subjects to treatment and control groups, the application of a variety of measuring instruments, and use of sophisticated statistical analysis to data thus gathered. While numerous studies using such approaches have been conducted, they have been criticized on methodological grounds, the narrow scope of behavior or personality being measured, and the inadequacy of the measuring instruments used.

At the present time, the area where advance is most likely to be made is in determining goals acceptable to most schools of psychotherapy and the further development and refinement of measuring instruments designed to assess patient progress toward these goals.

A survey of the evaluation literature reveals that six major strategies are currently used to assess community mental-health services, with some approaches offering a number of evaluation instruments from which to choose. There is, however, no agreement yet as to which are the best evaluation strategies or the most-useful measuring instruments within a particular approach.

After a brief description of the six main approaches to evaluation, and highlighting their major strengths and weaknesses, we shall describe the development, standardization, and heuristic value of a new instrument designed specifically for evaluating the impact of various community mental-health programs on the adaptive functioning of clients in the communities where they live.

Consumer Satisfaction Questionnaires

Consumer satisfaction questionnaires (CSQ) are designed to gauge the degree of clients' satisfaction with services rendered. The process usually entails mailing, telephoning, or interviewing clients at some point during treatment and/or after treatment ended. Consumer satisfaction with services influences the center's reputation in the community, thus affecting funding for new program requests and/or continuation of existing programs, which frequently need to demonstrate broad community support before submission or resubmission for funding. Furthermore, consumer satisfaction has an impact both on the number of referrals made to a mental-health center and the manner in which they are made. It also plays an important role in determining whether a therapeutic relationship is maintained, which is believed to be critical for successful problem solving and therefore favorable therapeutic outcome. Assessing consumer satisfaction is therefore recognized as important by most community mental-health-center programs. The advantages of the system lie in its simplicity of administration, low cost, and ease of data analysis.

The problem arises when, in lieu of other relevant data, community mental-health centers rely exclusively upon this source of information as indicative of their impact on clients served. The drawbacks of relying on this system of evaluation as a substitute for direct outcome studies are well known. Albers (1977) reviewed the literature on the subject of client satisfaction with services and found that response rate, irrespective of method used to encourage returns, usually does not exceed 30 percent. Our own studies confirm these findings (see appendix B). The likelihood of sampling bias makes the data gathered by CSQ studies difficult to interpret, particularly since dissatisfied clients are believed not to respond. Additionally, of those who respond to CSQ, their answers are believed to depend to a large degree on their perceived need for service upon initiation of therapy. Also frequently noted is that the interaction of satisfaction with service vis-à-vis satisfaction with outcome is uncertain. Most studies cited by Albers have found no clear relationship between satisfaction levels and quality of outcome. Although it is reasonable to expect that the client's understanding and acceptance of the therapist's role in the problem-solving process influences level of satisfaction, it is as yet uncertain to what degree and with what kind of clients. Furthermore, the yea-saying and social-desirability response sets (defined, respectively, as responding as one thinks one is expected to respond and a bias toward creating the impression of good mental health) are confounding variables in all consumer-satisfaction studies that we do not yet know how to partial out or control. Finally, consumer-satisfaction studies to gauge the effectiveness of programs do not enable us to determine how services help or fail to help a client, thus making the question of program improvement unanswerable.

Personality Inventories

The use of personality inventories as an evaluation strategy involves selecting a standardized, theoretically relevant inventory for a particular population and administering it before, during and/or after treatment. Typical examples include the use of Baron's Ego Strength Scale (Baron 1953) with psychotics, Taylor's Manifest Anxiety Scale (Taylor 1953) with neurotics, and Rotter's Internal-External Control Scale (Rotter 1966) with alcoholics. Since these scales purport to measure enduring personality traits, changes wrought along these dimensions are of great clinical importance and theoretical interest.

This approach to outcome evaluation has a number of drawbacks when applied to assessment of clients served by a community mental-health center. First, available evidence indicates that about two-thirds of all clients served in outpatient mental-health clinics are seen for fewer than ten sessions (for example, Garfield 1971: 275). This fact alone makes it highly unlikely that measurable changes in basic personality structure are, or can be, accomplished. Some of the more commonly used inventories, such as the Minnesota Multiphasic Personality Inventory, have been developed and standardized on patient populations using symptom clusters that discriminate among diagnostic groupings. Such standardization makes it unlikely that these instruments have the required sensitivity to tap gradual changes in personality dynamics, adjustment, or extent of psychopathology. Garfield, Prager, and Bergin (1971) is a case in point. They report that change scores on the MMPI were not related to client, therapist, or supervisor rating of improvements. Another difficulty is that for many pathological conditions treated in a community mental-health center (for example, gross immaturity, borderline conditions, sexual deviations), there are no standardized personality inventories. Finally, the proper collection and interpretion of data that personality inventories yield are exceedingly complex, expensive, and time-consuming to do for large groups, on a continual basis, which is essential for any meaningful program evaluation.

Improvement Ratings

Improvement ratings in broad areas of functioning are frequently relied upon to assess treatment outcome. Improved adjustment to family, work, or community or overall global functioning is rated on such scales by marking "improved," "somewhat improved," "no change," or "worse." The scoring is simple and requires minimal time and effort.

Reliance on this type of measurement, however, has certain limitations, particularly in interpretation of results. Interpretation of outcome is always uncertain, since each rater uses his or her own private standards and values for making the ratings. What is improved in the opinion of one therapist may be considered only somewhat improved by another; furthermore, the specific domain (for example, punctuality) selected for judgment by one therapist in such a global area as job adjustment may not be the same as that selected by another therapist (for example, acceptance by fellow employees). These differences make it difficult to compare and interpret the results obtained across therapists, treatment modalities, and programs. Unless a common frame of reference for such ratings is conceptualized, their meaning and value are uncertain at best. The current lack of a generally accepted frame of reference that is satisfactorily standardized is a major drawback of the various improvement-rating systems.

Symptom Checklists

Symptom checklists are usually easy to fill out and take little time to administer. Depending on the system selected, the checklist yields either one score or a number of subscores. Overall the method is considered useful for assessing short-term-crises intervention therapy that is designed to achieve symptomatic relief.

One of the chief disadvantages of the system is its reliance on the client's reporting of his or her subjective experience in relationship to the symptom. An "identical" symptomatic condition may be described by one client as very severe, yet another client may describe it as mild. Another important drawback is of a psychometric nature: most symptom checklists have a strong loading on one factor, which makes them of questionable value for differential interpretation in terms of symptom clusters. As far as outcome is concerned, reduction in symptomatology is only one of a number of goals of most systems of psychotherapy; the criteria required to judge improvement are much broader. These criteria should encompass (Strupp and Hadley 1977) the client's frame of reference ("feelings of well-being"), the significant other's point of view ("conformity to social codes"), and the therapist's judgment ("healthy personality"). Symptom checklists encompass too narrow a scope to represent adequately the goals of most schools of psychotherapy.

Goal Attainment Scaling

Goal-attainment scaling (GAS) requires that scales be developed individually for each client on the basis of his or her expressed problem areas. Progress is assessed against a series of positive and negative possible outcomes in the areas selected (Kiresuk and Sherman 1968). Levels of possible outcome are developed for each client from the least-favorable outcome expected to the most-likely level of outcome, through to the most-favorable outcome anticipated. Goals are stated in behavioral terms so that their attainment can be ascertained by an independent evaluator.

Information about a client's background, resources, level of motivation, and other factors can be taken into account in the process of goal setting. This system is unique in that outcome goals are tailored to the individual client in terms of that person's special clinical, personal, and social circumstances. Furthermore, the method has the advantage of giving direction to treatment and making therapists aware ahead of time what will be the basis upon which progress is to be assessed.

While the system of individual goal setting has great flexibility over more-structured methods of assessment, it has a number of unresolved problems of methodology, data analysis, and interpretation of results. At the present time very little is known about the process of negotiating goals with patients. Our own inquiry revealed that it is a much more complex undertaking than it appears. For example, the system is hard to apply meaningfully to clients who are not cooperative or are unduly argumentative. Another difficulty with this system lies in the selection of problems for scaling; it is uncertain which values or norms therapists use in this selection process. Another difficulty with the system is that a client's presenting complaint may be an expression of a broader personality difficulty. For example, a complaint around money management in a marriage might emanate from a sense of personal insecurity of one of the spouses, leading to distrust and control, through money, of the other spouse's independence. If the goal of better money management were achieved, the underlying insecurity may manifest itself through an even more destructive expression of suspicion or jealousy. Thus much skill and experience are required to select meaningful and conceptually independent problem areas and specify the behavior appropriate to the various scale steps. Thus, the scales chosen often vary considerably in quality and pertinence.

As far as statistical analysis is concerned, summarizing the data and arriving at a score is tedious and time-consuming. Furthermore application of standard statistical tests to pooled data is questionable, since the input consists of averages of different numbers of goals representing a more or less narrow range of items for each individual. Additionally interpretation of results in such a system is always problematic because the method, while emphasizing the uniqueness of each client, does not balance the selected goals against standard criteria of adjustment, which are essential for meaningful program evaluation. Consequently one is always forced to choose from among competing hypotheses since progress may reflect real improvement or more modest goals or healthier clients. Finally if the GAS technique is to be implemented routinely across all programs by all staff on a continuous basis, it requires a commitment of costly professional time to paperwork, which is usually unavailable in a clinical, nonresearch-oriented agency.

Measures of Personal, Social, and Community
Adjustment

Scales developed to measure personal, social, and community adjustment use either a client's responses to a questionnaire or a structured interview to obtain the required information (see, for example, Katz and Lyerly 1963; Endicott and Spitzer 1972; Ciarlo and Reihman 1974). Information from clients and significant others is usually obtained for the purpose of establishing level of functioning before treatment begins; the process is repeated at specified time intervals and/or at termination of therapy. The questionnaires usually have satisfactory reliability and some evidence that they assess what they purport to measure. Ciarlo and Reihman have introduced the novel idea of obtaining criterion data on persons in the community where the clients live to serve as ultimate goals of therapy. Although these measures appear to be more relevant, better standardized, and more comprehensive than other measures used for evaluating mental-health services, they have not yet demonstrated their value for improving decision making in the clinical area or in the broader domains of programming, administration, and policymaking.

From an economic standpoint, the routine administration of these scales is time-consuming; the cost of properly collecting and updating the information can be quite high. With some of these scales there is the problem of relying on significant others for information about adult clients. Such data gathering is fraught with clinical, ethical, and methodological problems. For example, obtaining the client's prior informed consent for interviewing relatives to obtain information about them and the client's privilege to refuse granting such consent raises questions about the generalizability of obtained results. Moreover, extensive clinical experience points against relying on the assumption that the reporting of significant others is sufficiently objective and impartial to be used as the sole criterion for judging outcome.

Summary

Each of the systems reviewed here is useful for certain purposes, but most have considerable limitations when applied to evaluating the impact of interventions on the broad array of clients served by community mental-health services.

This book will describe the development and standardization of a new instrument, the Progress Evaluation Scales (PES), which was designed to overcome many of the conceptual and technical problems noted in other evaluation approaches. A number of special studies, using a consumer satisfaction questionnaire, are described in appendix B.

Origins of the Progress Evaluation Scales

A number of important developments in the conceptualization and assessment of behavior change have influenced the construction of the PES scales. Particularly influential was the pioneering work of Kiresuk and Sherman (1968) on goal-attainment scaling. Their system of translating traditional clinical terminology into behavioral descriptions that lend themselves to quantitative analysis, as well as their method of establishing entry status and forecasting favorable and unfavorable therapy outcomes over specified time intervals, have influenced our thinking in major ways.

Another important influence on the construction of the PES was the work of Ciarlo and Reihman (1974), who advanced the idea that goals of therapy, as well as therapy outcome, should be set and measured against empirically established norms of functioning in the community where the scales are to be used.

A third major influence was the consensus that developed among all the participants in the project, irrespective of whether they viewed functioning from a dynamic, behavioristic, or structural frame of reference, that to be valid, a measure of adjustment needs to take into account both observable behavior and clients' subjective experience.

The fourth major influence on the development of the PES consisted of a series of clinical, administrative, and psychometric considerations that were found to be problematic in other assessment methodologies. Whether the PES is indeed free of similar drawbacks remains to be seen. Our effort focused on selecting dimensions for scaling that are relevant for clinical and programmatic decision making; developing administration procedures that are easy to follow yet unintrusive to the clinical process; adapting a computerized analysis system to minimize the need for extensive clerical resources, which otherwise would be needed and which most community mental-health centers can ill afford; exploring extensively such issues as therapist bias in use of the scales, the differences between long-term and short-term therapy goals when projected by therapists vis-à-vis clients, the advantages and disadvantages of using a narrow range (five-point) vis-à-vis an expanded scale (eleven points), and analyzing interrater agreement from a generalizability standpoint rather than the traditional correlational approach, which, while yielding higher coefficients, is actually less trustworthy for decision making since it does not take into account differences in the mean and variance of score distributions.

Description of the Progress Evaluation Scales

The PES are made up of seven scales, each consisting of five levels, with the characteristics of each level described. For statistical purposes, the five points in each scale have been assigned a value of 1 to 5, from the most pathological to the healthiest levels of functioning observed in the community. All seven scales are printed on a single page for ease of administration and handling. Four slightly different versions of the scales are available to accommodate children (ages 6 to 12), adolescents (ages 13 to 17), and adult mental-health clients and the developmentally disabled.

The seven dimensions of the PES were chosen to represent the major areas in which health and psychopathology reveal themselves. This selection was influenced by classical psychoanalytic theory and by other, more-recent studies of positive mental health. Two general propositions underlie the psychoanalytic conception of mental health. First, health and psychopathology are end points of a single continuum: "no sharp line can be drawn [between them] . . . our conception of 'disease' is purely . . . a matter of degree" (Freud 1909: 286). Second, the healthy end of this continuum is characterized by the presence of a "capacity for work and enjoyment" (Fenichel 1945: 581). This psychoanalytic conception of normality has been complemented more recently by a number of penetrating studies of positive mental health (such as Jahoda 1958; Offer and Sabshin 1966; Soddy and Ahrenfeldt 1967). Although none of these studies has taken issue with the two broad psychoanalytic propositions, they have clarified the importance of specific factors, such as meaningful personal relationships, positive self-regard, effective coping capacity, and modulated expression of affect, as essential ingredients for satisfactory personal, social, vocational, and familial adjustment.

Our selection and scaling of the PES dimensions reflect both the notion of a single continuum for health and psychopathology, as well as the consensus that has emerged in the professional literature concerning the areas that should be scrutinized for the presence of evidence of positive mental health and psychopathology.

Overall our focus was on measuring change toward healthy adaptive functioning rather than on relief of symptoms or personality reconstruction. This approach was selected since it appeared to approximate best the mandate of community mental-health centers. These centers, as do most other outpatient clinics, report consistently that over two-thirds of their clients are treated for fewer than ten sessions (Garfield 1971: 275). This fact alone makes the goal of achieving basic changes in the personality structure of most of these patients unlikely. Furthermore, while the majority of patients entering therapy usually focus their initial attention

on their symptoms and problems, most eventually realize that much of
their discomfort is due to faulty habits, unrealistic expectations, difficulties in establishing meaningful relationships, and the like; in the process of therapy they are led to recognize that if they are to bring about
lasting improvement in their problems, they may have to modify their
expectations, make changes in their life-style, and acquire more-effective
coping skills. The goals of therapy, as reflected by the high points of the
PES scales, are congruent both with recent findings on positive mental
health and with Freud's exhortation to his fellow practitioners to make
their therapeutic aim the "win[ning] back part of the capacity for work
and enjoyment" (Freud 1912: 332).

Descriptions of the scale points for the PES were developed with the
help of the clinical staff and suggestions from numerous patients, as well
as by empirical studies to determine score distribution, reliability, and
relationship among the various scales. The seven scales and the underlying
dimensions they represent follow.

Family Interaction

This scale measures the dimension of dependence-independence-interdependence in one's relationship with other family members. The lowest
level of functioning describes extreme dependent behavior where one
needs help with such basic needs as eating and dressing; in the middle
range one makes own plans and decisions but without necessarily considering the needs of other family members; at the highest level of functioning one plans and acts in such a manner that one's own needs, as
well as needs of others in the family, are taken into account.

Occupation (School-Job-Homemaking)

This scale taps a person's level of functioning in his or her primary
occupational role. At the lowest level of functioning, the person is unable
to hold a job, or care for home, or go to school; at the highest level of
functioning on this dimension, the person holds a regular job or attends
classes or carries out homemaker tasks (or some combination of these)
with little or no difficulty.

Getting Along with Others

This scale was designed to tap the dimension of socialization. The person's ability to establish and maintain satisfying relationships outside his
or her family circle is a reflection of the degree to which this kind of

socialization has satisfactorily occurred. The lowest level is characterized by a person who is always fighting, or is destructive, or is alone; the highest level characterizes a person who gets along with others most of the time and has close, regular friends. (This scale does not attempt to differentiate the hostile person from the recluse; both are considered equally unsocialized.)

Feelings and Mood

This scale taps the level of affective modulation as indicated by the degree to which feelings are flexibly expressed and adaptively integrated into overall personality functioning. At the least-satisfactory level of integration of affect, the person always feels nervous, depressed, angry or bitter or feels no emotions at all. The highest level of satisfactory affect integration is expressed in being in a good mood most of the time, as well as being able to be as happy or sad, or angry as the situation calls for. (Although the nature of affect at various levels is described, it is the persistence of certain affects that is measured.)

Use of Free Time

This scale assesses the degree to which sublimatory processes have satisfactorily evolved by indicating how free or constricted a person is in using inner and outer resources for play and enjoyment. The lowest level of functioning on this dimension is expressed in a person's almost total lack of interest in recreational activities or hobbies. The highest level of functioning is expressed in a person's participation in as well as ability to create a variety of own recreational activities and hobbies.

Problems

This scale taps the coping capacity the person can bring to bear on his or her daily problems. At the lowest level of functioning the person is unable to handle even mild problems; hence he or she experiences severe difficulties most of the time. At the highest level of functioning the individual is able to handle most situations well; therefore he or she is described as having only occasionally mild problems. ("Severe" refers to being incapacitated in important areas of adjustment, such as home-making, work, sex, communication, or parenting; "moderate" refers to being impaired in one's efficiency and/or effectiveness, but not totally incapacitated; "mild" refers to being "annoyed or inconvenienced" but not incapacitated or impaired in one's functioning in important areas).

Attitude toward Self

This scale assesses the dimension of self-esteem, in terms of the balance of negative and positive attitudes expressed about self. The lowest-level score is characterized as having a negative attitude toward self most of the time. The middle level is described as having an almost equal positive and negative attitude toward self. The highest level is characterized as having a positive attitude toward self most of the time.

To use the scales, therapists, clients, and/or significant others independently indicate the initial status of clients by selecting the one item in each scale that describes best their current functioning level. "Current functioning" is defined as typical behavior and experience during two weeks preceding the evaluation interview.

After current status is indicated on one sheet for the seven scales of the PES, goals are set on a different sheet, again independently by therapists, clients, and/or significant others. For adults who can read at the level of comprehending a daily newspaper article, the clients themselves and their therapists do the rating. For adults unable to read or who are too disturbed to perform this task satisfactorily themselves, therapists and significant others perform the ratings. For children and adolescents, therapists and significant others perform the ratings. Adolescents are encouraged to do an additional rating of their own.

For outpatient services, three-month goals are set initially, with new six-month goals set at each review period thereafter for as long as clients are in treatment. When the case is closed (three months after no contact with the clinic), a closing rating is made by the therapist. At this time, patients are mailed a rating form and are requested to return it with their self-evaluation. For clients enrolled in rehabilitation programs (such as, day treatment or a sheltered workshop), where some progress is expected in the vocational, social, or personal domains, initial and subsequent goals are set on a six-months' basis. For clients in maintenance programs (such as day activities), where minimal progress is expected and where the goals are defined more in terms of containment of psychopathology and support of current functioning levels in the community, initial and subsequent goals are set on a twelve-months' basis.

Clinicians who are familiar with the scales can fill them out in a minute or two at the end of the diagnostic interview. Patients and significant others, whose reading level is that of being able to comprehend a daily newspaper, can fill out the scale in five to eight minutes.

Over eight years, numerous studies were conducted utilizing the PES with various patient samples in order to answer questions such ease of use, clarity of language, and ordering and spacing of behavioral descriptions for each dimension. Additionally, data were collected to help determine the more-quantitative psychometric properties of the scales, such as score distribution, rater reliability, similarities and differences in rating of therapist, patient, and significant other, sex and age differences in ratings, normative group ratings, and the like. Since the scale *Attitude toward Self* was the last to be developed, somewhat less information is available on it than on the other six scales.

Preliminary Studies

Some of the preliminary studies involved in the development of the PES may be useful to those planning to utilize the scales with any of the targeted populations. Detailed instructions for administering the PES are given in appendix A.

Examination of Therapist Bias

One of the first areas investigated was the possibility of bias in the use of scales by different therapists. We wondered whether there might be a tendency for some therapists to score patients consistently higher or lower on certain scales than did other therapists. In an attempt to examine this question, average ratings were determined on 25 patients from each of six therapists, plus fewer patients from two additional therapists. Since patients were not randomly assigned, the best way to examine these ratings is by comparing differences between patients' and therapists' ratings for each scale. Of course, this method would also be invalid if the selection of patients tends to augment this difference for some groups. For example, many alcoholics are known to deny problems and claim all is well with them. Thus a therapist seeing a large number of alcoholics might rate patients considerably lower, on the average, than they rate themselves.

   In general our results indicate that average ratings of patient and therapist for initial status and goals were quite close—67 percent of them lying within 0.25 points of each other. However, several rather large differences were noted. The largest, 0.92, occurred for one therapist on status ratings of *Use of Free Time*. This therapist rated higher, on the average, than did his clients, whereas two other therapists had ratings averaging 0.52 and 0.58 lower than their clients. Thus, there was a total swing of 1.5 points. It appeared, therefore, that there was a serious difficulty in the interpretation of this scale. Further questioning and discussion revealed considerable uncertainty regarding interpretation of scale levels, resulting in a change in the description of some of the scale points. This change was incorporated into the next revision.

Another large discrepancy occurred on the scale *Feelings and Mood* for two therapists. Both therapists rated their patients consistently lower on initial status than the patients rated themselves. Furthermore, although therapists generally tended to set lower goals than did patients, their goal ratings on this scale showed the largest differences. These discrepancies were discussed with the staff, with the result that further modifications were made in the descriptions of the scale points.

Open-Ended versus Three-Month Goals

In the first year in which the PES scales were used, no time period was specified with regard to goal setting. The instruction stated simply, "Indicate how you expect to be at the end of counseling." The goals set under these instructions (generally falling at the 4 or 5 level on all scales) seemed considerably higher than one might reasonably expect for outpatient mental-health clients in short-term therapy. We decided, therefore, to determine what effect would result from specifying a fixed period of time: three months. These instructions were used during the second year.

Samples of adults and adolescents were drawn from patients seen in each year, selecting only those who had self-ratings and ratings of significant others as well as therapist ratings. Samples of children who were rated by both parent and therapist were also compared. The summary data for these samples are displayed in tables 1–1, 1–2, and 1–3. Data in these tables pertain to only six scales. The seventh scale, *Attitude toward Self,* had not yet been developed.

Ratings of present status were similar whether made by therapist, patient, or significant other for adults seen the first year (table 1–1). The average goal ratings, with one or two exceptions, were also similar when the target time was not specified. In fact, patients and significant others had almost identical means, with the largest difference (0.12) occurring for *Feelings and Mood.* For this variable, the therapists' goals were significantly lower than were those of the patient or the significant other. The therapists also set a lower goal, on the average, for the *Problems* scale. However, for therapist, patient, and significant other, goals were set at a fairly constant distance above ratings for present status, averaging 1.34, 1.40, and 1.38, respectively, over the six scales.

In the second sample (three-month goals) the ratings of therapist and patient differed both with regard to present functioning and to goals. (Differences in present status are not significant but are large enough to obscure the effect of a change in instructions on goal setting.) The goal

Table 1–1
Means and Standard Deviations for PES Ratings of Therapist, Patient, and Significant Other in Two Adult Outpatient Samples

| | Sample 1: Open-ended Goals (N = 33) | | | | | | Sample 2: Three-Month Goals (N = 35) | | | | | |
| | Therapist | | Patient | | Other | | Therapist | | Patient | | Other | |
Scale	X̄	sd	X̄	sd	X̄	sd	X̄	sd	X̄·	sd	X̄	sd
Family Interaction												
Present	3.55	1.00	3.61	1.03	3.52	1.06	3.66	0.64	3.77	0.91	3.69	1.11
Goal	4.70	.47	4.76	.71	4.67	.89	4.29	.67	4.74	.56	4.80	.41
Occupation												
Present	3.94	1.37	4.00	1.25	3.94	1.32	3.71	1.34	3.80	1.35	3.69	1.39
Goal	4.73	.63	4.73	.57	4.79	.55	4.51	.56	4.86	.43	4.77	.49
Getting Along with Others												
Present	3.55	.97	3.67	1.11	3.70	1.05	3.49	.89	4.14	.85	3.80	.96
Goal	4.42	.71	4.55	.75	4.45	.83	4.11	.72	4.43	.74	4.69	.47
Feelings and Mood												
Present	2.67	1.11	2.88	1.34	2.85	1.30	2.83	.18	3.37	1.24	3.23	1.26
Goal	4.36	.78	4.76	.66	4.64	.65	4.09	.78	4.69	.68	4.83	.38
Use of Free Time												
Present	2.55	1.10	2.76	1.62	2.67	1.41	2.83	1.07	3.34	1.30	2.91	1.20
Goal	4.36	.70	4.33	1.19	4.36	1.08	3.97	.82	4.54	.74	4.34	.97
Problems												
Present	2.45	.71	2.52	1.33	2.58	1.32	2.71	.96	2.71	1.10	3.11	1.18
Goal	4.27	.63	4.70	.68	4.61	.70	3.83	.75	4.40	.85	4.63	.49

Table 1-2
Progress Evaluation Ratings of Adolescents by Patient, Therapist, and Significant Other

| | Sample 1: Open-ended goals (N = 18) | | | | | | Sample 2: Three-Month Goals (N = 18) | | | | | |
| | Therapist | | Patient | | Other | | Therapist | | Patient | | Other | |
Scale	X̄	sd	X̄	sd	X̄	sd	X̄	sd	X̄	sd	X̄	sd
Family Interaction												
Present	3.56	0.98	3.56	1.10	3.33	1.08	4.00	0.76	3.87	1.12	3.73	0.96
Goal	4.56	.62	4.61	.50	4.50	.86	4.53	.52	4.47	.64	4.47	.64
Occupation												
Present	3.33	.84	3.28	1.02	3.22	1.11	3.53	.99	3.47	.83	3.53	1.19
Goal	4.56	.51	4.72	.57	4.61	.61	4.20	.86	4.07	.80	4.33	.98
Getting Along with Others												
Present	3.56	.70	4.06	.80	3.67	1.24	3.87	1.12	4.20	.94	3.93	1.03
Goal	4.56	.51	4.83	.38	4.61	.98	4.20	.94	4.73	.46	4.27	.88
Feelings and Mood												
Present	3.56	.78	3.50	.86	3.39	1.29	2.87	.99	3.87	1.19	3.73	1.16
Goal	4.67	.48	4.72	.57	4.83	.51	4.20	.77	4.53	.64	4.47	.99
Use of Free Time												
Present	3.61	1.04	3.44	1.20	3.06	1.59	3.67	1.05	3.93	.80	3.40	1.06
Goal	4.61	.50	4.67	.59	4.67	.59	4.27	.70	4.20	.94	4.27	.96
Problems												
Present	3.33	.68	3.67	.84	3.22	.81	2.80	.68	3.53	.83	3.07	.88
Goal	4.67	.48	4.89	.32	4.61	.50	3.87	.64	4.33	.82	4.20	.94

Table 1–3
Progress Evaluation Ratings of Children by Parent and Therapist

| | Sample 1: Open-ended Goals (N = 30) | | | | Sample 2: Three-Month Goals (N = 18) | | | |
| | Parent | | Therapist | | Parent | | Therapist | |
Scale	X̄	sd	X̄	sd	X̄	sd	X̄	sd
Family Interaction								
Present	2.97	1.27	3.47	1.31	3.72	1.02	4.06	0.80
Goal	4.50	.82	4.60	.72	4.28	.75	4.61	.50
Occupation								
Present	3.27	1.41	3.30	1.24	3.94	1.00	3.94	1.00
Goal	4.40	.97	4.30	.88	4.61	.61	4.39	.70
Getting Along with Others								
Present	3.10	1.27	3.57	1.01	2.94	.87	3.39	1.09
Goal	4.67	.55	4.63	.49	4.00	.68	4.28	.67
Feelings and Mood								
Present	3.40	1.30	3.33	1.32	3.06	1.39	3.11	.90
Goal	4.83	.46	4.77	.43	4.56	.62	4.33	.77
Use of Free Time								
Present	3.63	1.03	3.73	1.11	3.00	1.14	3.33	.84
Goal	4.77	.43	4.63	.49	4.17	.86	4.28	.75
Problems								
Present	2.97	1.22	3.20	.92	3.33	.69	3.33	.59
Goal	4.76	.43	4.57	.50	4.33	.59	4.33	.59

ratings of the therapists appeared lowered relative to sample 1, as might realistically be expected. The drop ranged from 0.22 for *Occupation* to 0.44 for *Problems*. The average difference between present status ratings and goal ratings dropped forty-one units, from 1.34 to 0.93. The goal ratings of patients and significant others did not appear much different from those set by the sample with open-ended goals. However, when the data were examined in terms of the average difference between present status and goals, a decrease was again noted. The drop for patients averaged 0.31, while that for significant others was only 0.14.

Comparing the mean ratings for adolescents in the two samples (table 1–2), one finds that while the patients on the second sample (short-term goals) rated themselves higher on initial status for five of the first six scales than did the first sample, they set lower goals on all six scales. The average differences between initial status and goal ratings were 1.16 for open-ended goals and 0.58 for three-month goals. A similar drop in goals relative to initial-status ratings occurred for the parents; the average difference dropped from 1.32 to 0.66. In this respect, they both rated similarly to the therapists who also tended to set goals closer to initial status when three months were specified. Thus, there is no evidence of unrealistic goal setting for these samples of adolescents or their parents.

The ratings by parent and therapist for two small groups of children were also analyzed (table 1–3). Again, one group (N = 30) indicated open-ended goals, while the second (N = 18) set three-month goals. With one or two exceptions, therapists characterized the children as better adjusted than did the parents. On the other hand, the goals set by parents and therapists were quite close to each other in both samples. Looking again at the difference between status and goal ratings, that for the therapist dropped from 1.15 in the sample with open-ended goals to 0.84 in the sample with three-month goals. The corresponding mean differences for the parent were 1.43 and 0.99, respectively.

From these data it was evident that therapists, patients, and parents all adjust their goals when instructed to project them for a specified time interval as compared to their goals for the vaguely defined end of therapy. Only the ratings of the patient's spouse failed to respond realistically to the difference in instructions. Since *termination of therapy* is a vague concept and in many cases not particularly meaningful in view of the fact that about two-thirds of outpatient mental-health clients discontinue therapy within a three-month period, it was decided that three-month goals would be set for all outpatients. At the end of three months the patient would be reevaluated and if still in therapy, new goals would be set for the next six months.

A further decision arising from these data and other considerations was that ratings would no longer be obtained from spouses of adult outpatients. One of the major reasons for this decision was an ethical one regarding the patients' right to object to having their spouses rate them. It was also found that in some cases the patient would agree to this procedure only if he or she could see the spouse's ratings. This necessitated informing the spouse that the ratings would not be kept confidential. The problems thus raised both with regard to the validity of such data and to the therapeutic management of the issue made the procedure undesirable both from the administrative and clinical standpoints.

Expanding the Scale

It was thought that the employment of an eleven-point scale, obtained by permitting the rater to use points midway between each behavioral description plus one below the lowest and above the highest description on the PES might increase the discriminating power of the scales. Consequently this scaling was attempted for fifty sequentially drawn adult mental-health clients. There was some difficulty in explaining to the clients how to utilize the eleven-point scale, but most of them seemed able to handle it satisfactorily.

An examination of the data showed that the expanded scale provided no apparent advantages insofar as rating present status. This conclusion was based on the following observations:

1. The mean scores for present status as rated by therapists and patients on the expanded scale were almost identical to those found in other samples on which the five-point scales were used when the appropriate scale transformation was employed to make them comparable.
2. The standard deviations were also approximately equivalent.
3. Correlations between ratings of therapists and patients were equal to or slightly lower than those of previous samples.
4. The intercorrelations among the separate scales as rated by therapist or by patient were higher than those obtained previously, indicating less differentiation among dimensions.

There were two indicators of some slight advantage of the expanded scale for expressing goals:

1. The standard deviations were somewhat larger than those on the five-point scale data, after correcting for the difference in number of intervals. This indicated greater individual differences in goal ratings.
2. There were significant negative correlations between age and patient goals on four of the seven scales. This relationship between goal setting and age had occurred in previous samples only for males on one scale: *Problems*. This finding could imply improved discrimination, but it could also have arisen as a result of sampling.

In conclusion, it appears that for the purposes intended—as a method of evaluating the effectiveness of programs for groups of people—the present five-point scales are adequate. For more-precise evaluation of individuals and for statistical analysis employing parametric assumptions, it might be better to provide scales with finer discriminations such as the eleven-point scale used in this study. Further exploration of such scales would be necessary prior to their use.

Reliability versus Generalizability

An important consideration in the development of any measurement instrument and procedure is the extent to which scores are generalizable to the universe they are intended to represent. Most test manuals deal with this issue in terms of reliability. Questions of agreement among raters, stability over time, and internal consistency among items are examined separately in each case by obtaining two sets of scores and computing the correlation between them. While this method may be appropriate for paper-and-pencil tests that approximately meet the assumptions of classical psychometric theory, they ignore many of the problems involved in rating scales. In particular, it cannot be assumed that different raters generate scales with the same distributions with respect to their means and variance. Furthermore, in the actual employment of rating scales by therapists, a different therapist interviews and rates each client. Thus, differences in style of interview as well as differences in rating affect the resulting scores and contribute to their unreliability in assessing individual differences among clients. Correlations disregard these differences. Cronbach and his associates (1972) have developed a theory of generalizability to deal with this problem. Their approach attempts to isolate and estimate components of variance attributable to various aspects of the measuring procedure, thus making it possible to estimate the error variance of scores as they will be used in the decision situation. For some purposes a coefficient of generalizability indicating the proportion of observed variance attributable to true variance is meaningful. Such coefficients are somewhat lower than the reliability coefficients usually presented for rating scales and assessment instruments, but they more realistically represent the confidence that can be placed in an obtained score.

A number of problems are encountered in obtaining estimates of generalizability for rating procedures. One is that it is almost impossible to obtain estimates of variance over interviewers on the same client. Scheduling two interviews for a client by different interviewers in close succession to cover the same questions is theoretically possible, but practically it is likely to interfere considerably with the operation of a busy mental-health center as well as imposing on the client and endangering the necessary therapeutic alliance between client and therapist. A second problem is encountered in determining stability of ratings over time. Since the PES scales are measures of the state of adjustment of the client, they cannot be expected to yield the same scores if the client is in a state of flux. Furthermore, it is change of the client over time that the scales are intended to tap. Yet, certainly, the scale levels allude to behaviors that are typical over some short period of time. We have arbitrarily set this period as two weeks. However, any estimate of the stability of the resulting scale ratings will confound client instability with rater instability and hence be an underestimate of the stability of ratings per se.

Since PES scales are usually filled out by both therapist and client, one could consider such ratings as interchangeable. If this generalization were intended, differences in ratings between therapist and client would also be a source of error. We have chosen, however, to treat ratings of therapist and client as representative of two different viewpoints or perceptions and, hence, as separate, albeit related, variables. For the client's ratings there can be no universe of raters; this aspect of the rating is fixed. However, setting and occasion of rating are sources of error, and difference in clients' understanding of directions and rating style affects the variance of scores across clients, thus serving to reduce the correlation between client and therapist.

2

Application of Progress Evaluation Scales to Adult Populations

Generalizability Studies

Agreement among Therapists

An early study carried out with these scales was designed to determine to what extent therapists differ in their assessment of current status of individual clients and in setting goals for therapy. For this purpose a staff member sat in on the initial interview by the therapist and independently rated the client as to present status and three-month goals. A sample of 20 adults were rated in this fashion. Data for only the first six scales are available, since the seventh scale, *Attitude toward Self,* had not yet been developed.

The mean profiles for clients as rated by two staff members are reported in table 2–1 and shown in figure 2–1. It is evident that with the exception of one or two scales, the current-status profiles are in close agreement. The largest difference is 0.40 on the scales for *Family Inter-action* and *Use of Free Time.* These differences are not statistically significant, but they should not be dismissed in estimating therapist agreement. Average goal ratings are all quite close.

The data were analyzed for each scale separately to obtain estimates of the amount of variance attributable to differences among clients ($\hat{\sigma}_p^2$) and that due to average differences between ratings of therapists on any one person ($\hat{\sigma}_e^2$). The ratio of ($\hat{\sigma}_p^2$) to the expected observed-score variance ($\hat{\sigma}_x^2$) yields an estimate of reliability (r_{xx}). These values are also shown in table 2–1. This method of computing reliability takes into account the fact that in ordinary use of this scale, clients will be rated by different therapists. Therefore, therapist mean-score differences will contribute to both observed score and error variance. Such estimates, however, tend to be lower than those obtained by correlating the two sets of scores since the latter method ignores differences among therapists' means. Reliability estimates for current status ranged from 0.49 for *Problems* to a high of 0.86 for *Getting Along with Others.* The range of reliability for goals was somewhat lower (0.39 to 0.67). The median reliabilities were 0.65 for present status and 0.43 for goals.

Since reliability estimates depend heavily on the amount of variability

Table 2–1
Comparison of Two Therapists' Ratings on an Adult Outpatient Sample (N = 20)

Scale	Present Status						Goal Rating					
	M_{t_1}	M_{t_2}	$\hat{\sigma}^2_x$	$\hat{\sigma}^2_p$	$\hat{\sigma}^2_e$	r_{xx}	M_{t_1}	M_{t_2}	$\hat{\sigma}^2_x$	$\hat{\sigma}^2_p$	$\hat{\sigma}^2_e$	r_{xx}
Family Interaction	3.90	3.50	0.53	0.33	0.20	0.62	4.35	4.40	0.45	0.18	0.28	0.39
Occupation	4.30	4.35	.54	.37	.18	.68	4.75	4.75	.20	.10	.10	.49
Getting Along with Others	3.50	3.40	1.05	.90	.15	.86	4.05	4.15	.67	.45	.22	.67
Feelings and Mood	2.85	2.80	1.32	.79	.52	.60	4.05	3.95	.53	.18	.35	.34
Use of Free Time	3.40	3.00	1.68	1.28	.40	.76	4.05	3.95	1.04	.49	.55	.47
Problems	3.15	3.00	.64	.32	.32	.49	4.15	3.95	.41	.16	.25	.39

Note: M_{t_1} = mean for therapist 1. M_{t_2} = mean for therapist 2.
$\hat{\sigma}^2_x = \hat{\sigma}^2_p + \hat{\sigma}^2_e$.

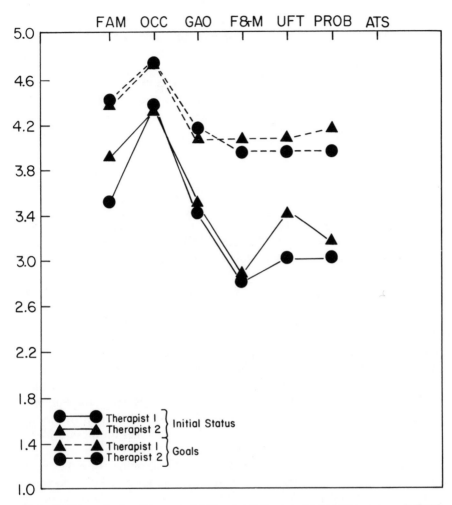

Note: In this and other figures and tables the following abbreviations are used: FAM = Family Interaction; OCC = Occupation; GAO = Getting Along with Others; F&M = Feelings and Mood; UFT = Use of Free Time; PROB = Problems; ATS = Attitude toward Self

Figure 2–1. Comparison of Two Therapists' Ratings for Initial Status and Goals for a Sample of Twenty Adult Outpatients

among subjects in the sample, a somewhat better idea of the extent to which ratings of a client might differ from one therapist to another is obtained from consideration of the estimates of error variance. For ratings of current status, these range from a high of 0.52 to a low of 0.15, with a mean of 0.30. Furthermore, although the reliability estimates for goals are lower than for current status, the estimates of error variance are in the same range, also averaging 0.30. These estimates imply that 90 percent of the time, therapists' ratings of an individual on these scales will lie within 0.9 unit from that obtainable were a large number of therapists to make every rating. Since the resolving power of the scale is one unit, this value does not appear unreasonably large. Furthermore, a difference of 0.4 between observed means of two groups of as few as ten clients, each rated by different therapists, is reliable at the 90 percent level of confidence.

Stability over Occasions

Stability of ratings over occasions was also examined. Sixty-five adult patients attending group-therapy sessions filled out rating scales on two occasions, two weeks apart. The therapist also rated them on both occasions. The estimated variance components resulting from this study are shown in table 2–2.

One result is quite clear: there is little, if any, systematic variance attributable to occasions of rating on any of the scales, or any differential trend over occasions between ratings of client and therapist (raters × occasions). Some differential trends over time are indicated for subjects (subject × occasions), particularly for *Use of Free Time, Feelings and Mood,* and *Problems,* all of which could legitimately be considered as scales measuring somewhat-transient states. The triple interaction, which includes all residual random error, is also relatively large for *Feelings and Mood* and *Use of Free Time.* Thus, therapist and client differ in the way their ratings change from one occasion to another on these scales.

At the bottom of table 2–2, the expected "true" score and error variances are computed under the assumption that ratings of either therapists or clients will be used exclusively and no generalization to other raters is intended. The reliability coefficient gives some indication of the stability of such ratings over occasions. Error variance ranged from 0.16 to 0.37, with a mean of 0.22. The coefficients of generalizability over occasions for present status ranged from 0.54 for *Family Interaction* to 0.75 for *Problems,* with a median of 0.68. For goals, the range was 0.44 to 0.62, with a median of 0.53. One deduction that can be made from these data is that a difference of one unit on a scale rated by the same therapist on two occasions represents a real change at the 90 percent level of confidence.

A comparison of the estimated variance for these clients with that in table 2–1 indicates that the present sample has a very restricted variance on the first scale, compared to a more-random sample of clients. If one were to use the estimated variance for clients obtained in the first sample,

Table 2–2
Estimates of Variance Components for Subject, Rater, Occasions of Rating, and Their Interaction Based on Sixty-Five Adult Clients in Group Therapy

| | Variance Estimates | | | | | | | | | | | |
| | Family Interaction | | Occupation | | Getting Along | | Feelings and Mood | | Use of Free Time | | Problems | |
Source	Present	Goal	Present	Goal	Present	Goal	Present	Goal	Present	Goal	Present	Goal
Subject	0.09	0.07	0.15	0.02	0.23	0.05	0.29	0.06	0.18	0.12	0.25	0.09
Rater	.01	.05	.00	.01	.06	.08	.02	.18	.00	.20	.00	.14
Occasion	.00	.00	.00	.00	.00	.00	.01	.00	.00	.00	.03	.00
Subject × rater	.10	.05	.19	.12	.21	.13	.36	.14	.36	.09	.28	.19
Subject × occupation	.01	.01	.01	.00	.01	.01	.04	.00	.11	.00	.03	.03
Rater × occupation	.00	.00	.00	.00	.00	.01	.00	.00	.00	.01	.00	.00
Subject × rater × occupation	.15	.14	.16	.12	.16	.13	.25	.18	.26	.27	.15	.14

For ratings obtained either from the therapist or the client, stability is estimated as

	Present	Goal	Present	Goal	Present	Goal	Present	Goal	Present	Goal	Present	Goal
Client ($\hat{\sigma}_p^2$)	.19	.12	.34	.14	.44	.18	.65	.20	.54	.21	.53	.28
$\hat{\sigma}_e^2$	.16	.15	.17	.12	.17	.15	.29	.18	.37	.27	.18	.17
r_α	.54	.44	.67	.54	.72	.55	.69	.53	.59	.44	.75	.62

the coefficient of stability would be 0.67, which is more in line with the coefficients obtained for the other scales. Using the same reasoning, the coefficient for the *Use of Free Time* scale may also be somewhat attenuated.

Combining the information about variance among raters from table 2–1 with the estimates of variance over occasions from table 2–2 yields estimates of the variance of therapists' ratings for a universe of raters and occasions of rating over a two-week period. These values range from 0.32 to 0.81, with a mean of 0.52 for the initial six scales. From these data we can deduce that 90 percent of the time a therapist's ratings on these scales will lie within 1.2 units from that obtainable were a large number of therapists to make ratings on the same individual within a two-week interval. If higher generalizability is desirable for a particular use, such as individual assessment, it can be obtained by averaging ratings of two therapists, made on separate occasions; this will reduce the 90 percent confidence interval to ± 0.8.

Goal Setting by Therapists

An interesting by-product of our study of the agreement among ratings of therapists is the relationship between the goals set by one therapist and the status ratings of another therapist. This can be distinguished from the correlations usually obtained between the status and goal ratings of a single therapist. These latter ratings contain correlated errors of measurement since they are made by the same individual at approximately the same time. Such correlations have been designated as linked by Cronbach et al. (1972) to distinguish them from correlations that do not share common conditions and hence are independent.

The linked and independent correlations between status and goal ratings for pairs of therapist-raters on 20 adults are displayed in table 2–3. As expected, the linked correlations are higher than the independent correlations for all scales, indicating the extent to which errors of measurement for current functioning and goals are interdependent. The unlinked correlations range from 0.23 for *Occupation* to 0.76 for *Getting Along With Others,* with a median of 0.38. They indicate a significant relationship between the status of a client and the goals that he or she might be expected to accomplish in a three-month period. A better indication of this relationship would be the correlation between error-free ratings, which are estimated in the last column of table 2–3. These correlations, which have been corrected for attenuation, indicate a very close relationship between client status and goals for three-month therapy for all but *Occupation.* It is very likely that this relationship is low because

Table 2–3
Correlations between Current Status and Three-Month Goals as Rated by Two Therapists for an Adult Psychiatric Sample (N = 20)

Scale	Same Rater (Linked)	Different Raters (Independent)	r Corrected for Attenuation
Family Interaction	0.48	0.40	0.82
Occupation	.51	.23	.40
Getting Along with Others	.84	.76	1.00
Feelings and Mood	.48	.33	.73
Use of Free Time	.79	.55	.92
Problems	.48	.36	.82

to a great extent occupational status was determined by factors outside the control of the therapist, particularly at the time these ratings were made, which was a period of high unemployment.

Construct Validity Studies

Comparison of Central Tendencies and Deviations from the Mean for Normative and Patient Populations

Means and Standard Deviations for Nonpatient Samples: The PES scales were constructed to evaluate clients' level of adjustment to family, job, and community, as well as their personal functioning. An implication of such scaling is that members of the community requiring no special services would obtain higher scores on these scales than would those who are emotionally disturbed. Thus, as Ciarlo and Reihman (1974) did, one might use the typical profiles of persons in the community as defining norms of adjustment, the ultimate goals of therapy. To test such an assumption, a sample of male and female adults from nonpatient populations was obtained. The adults males, 90 in all, were workers in a factory (31), PTA fathers (44), and graduate students (15). The females (171) were PTA mothers (88), gainfully employed nonprofessional women (34), professional women (24), and graduate-social-work students (25).

Three other nonpatient samples have been obtained, primarily to determine the sensitivity of the PES scales to differences in the population sampled. These groups consisted of 44 females from a Planned Parenthood clinic and male and female physically handicapped Goodwill workers (N = 17 and 31, respectively). The latter groups ranged in age from

18 to 67 and suffered from a wide range of disabilities, such as ampu-
tations, paralyses, heart disease, diabetes, and epilepsy. Educationally,
they ranged from eight grades or less to college graduates. The females
attending the Planned Parenthood clinic had a much more restricted age
range (16 to 40).

The means and standard deviations of self-ratings for these nonpatient
groups are shown in table 2–4. Typically all groups rate themselves
higher on the first four scales than on the last three. Adult females rate
themselves somewhat higher on *Family Interaction* than do males but
significantly lower on *Use of Free Time* and *Attitude toward Self.*

The physically handicapped subjects see themselves as being somewhat poorer on *Family Interaction* and *Occupation* than do the subjects
from the Planned Parenthood clinic or the normative sample. Both sexes
differ significantly ($p < 0.05$) from the normative sample on *Occupation,*
while the difference on *Family Interaction,* although equally large in both
samples, is statistically significant only for females. Additionally both
male and female physically handicapped rate themselves lower on *Use
of Free Time* than do the normative groups (males, $p < 0.05$, females,
$p < 0.01$). The women attending a Planned Parenthood clinic differ at the
0.05 level from the female normative group on *Getting Along with Others*
and *Problems* and at the 0.01 level on *Feelings and Mood, Use of Free
Time,* and *Attitude toward Self.*

These data yield important evidence of the validity of the PES as a
measure of community adjustment. Self-ratings on all seven scales re-
sulted in some meaningful discriminations among subgroups of the non-
psychiatric population. Ten of 28 comparisons were significant at or
beyond the 0.05 level despite the fact that the smallest group (the male
physically handicapped) consisted of only 17 subjects. Furthermore, all
differences were in the expected direction.

Means and Standard Deviations for Patient Samples: Over the years a
number of samples of outpatient ratings have been collected from the
Shiawassee Mental Health Center. For the present purposes, however,
it will suffice to examine means and standard deviations of self-ratings
on a sample of 50 males and 50 females seen in 1975 and samples of 111
males and 159 females seen in 1977 (table 2–5). Only the last two samples
rated themselves on the seventh scale, *Attitude toward Self.* Further data
on these samples will be given in subsequent sections of this book. Table
2–5 shows that with respect to both means and standard deviations, the
self-ratings of patients are extremely stable from one year to another. The
only scales on which they differ significantly in mean score are *Getting
Along with Others,* on which males seen in 1977 are higher, and *Occupation,* on which females seen in 1977 are higher than those seen in

Table 2–4
Means and Standard Deviations of PES Status Ratings for Nonpatient Adult Samples

Sample		Age	Family Interaction	Occupation	Getting Along with Others	Feelings and Mood	Use of Free Time	Problems	Attitude toward Self
Normative males (N = 90)	X̄	31.2	4.65	4.84	4.73	4.69	4.31	4.36	4.38
	sd	11.7	.60	.38	.45	.53	.90	.77	.74
Physically handicapped males (N = 17)	X̄	32.5	4.18	3.94[a]	4.29	4.47	3.35[a]	4.05	4.06
	sd	12.1	1.07	1.43	.99	1.01	1.62	.97	.90
Normative females (N = 171)	X̄	31.6	4.78	4.79	4.69	4.59	3.90	4.34	4.12
	sd	9.3	.51	.52	.55	.66	.93	.73	.99
Planned Parenthood females (N = 44)	X̄	24.2	4.61	4.57	4.39[a]	4.16[b]	3.34[b]	4.00[a]	3.66[b]
	sd	6.2	.62	.97	.72	.91	1.14	.89	.99
Physically handicapped females (N = 31)	X̄	38.3	4.38[a]	4.35[a]	4.48	4.29	3.26[b]	4.32	3.90
	sd	15.3	1.02	1.02	.62	1.04	1.26	.75	.83

[a] Significantly different from normative sample (Dunnett's multiple comparison procedure $p < 0.05$.)
[b] Ibid. $p < 0.01$.

Table 2–5
Means and Standard Deviations of Self-Ratings of Initial Status of Male and Female Outpatients

Sample		Age	Family Interaction	Occupation	Getting Along with Others	Feelings and Mood	Use of Free Time	Problems	Attitude toward Self
Males 1975 (N = 50)	X̄	30.4	3.94	4.06	3.70[b]	3.46	3.02	2.84	2.73
	sd	8.6	.84	1.17	.86	1.15	1.25	1.09	1.14
Males 1977 (N = 110)	X̄	34.1	3.85	4.01	4.08[b]	3.18	2.72	2.73	
	sd	12.2	.88	1.30	.92	1.28	1.36	1.20	
Females 1975 (N = 50)	X̄	34.5	3.94	3.88[a]	4.14	2.94	2.96	2.72	
	sd	12.5	.89	1.12	.83	1.18	1.34	1.03	
Females 1977 (N = 159)	X̄	31.5	4.13	4.21[a]	4.14	3.12	2.85	2.83	2.48
	sd	10.8	.71	.85	.90	1.20	1.52	1.05	1.03

[a] Significantly different, $p = 0.05$.
[b] Significantly different, $p = 0.05$.

1975. Those mean changes that occurred, however, are in the direction of eliminating all sex differences. Thus, in the 1975 samples, males reported poorer adjustment than did females on *Getting Along with Others* and better adjustment on *Feelings and Mood*. There are no sex differences in the later sample. Males and females from both years have a similar spread of scores, as indicated by the standard deviations.

Comparison of Patient and Nonpatient Samples: The scores for the 1977 patient sample are graphed in figures 2–2 and 2–3, together with the

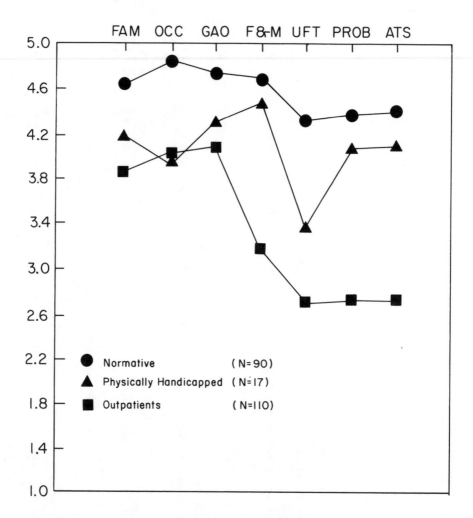

Figure 2–2. Comparison of Self-Ratings of Normative, Physically Handicapped Males and Outpatient Males

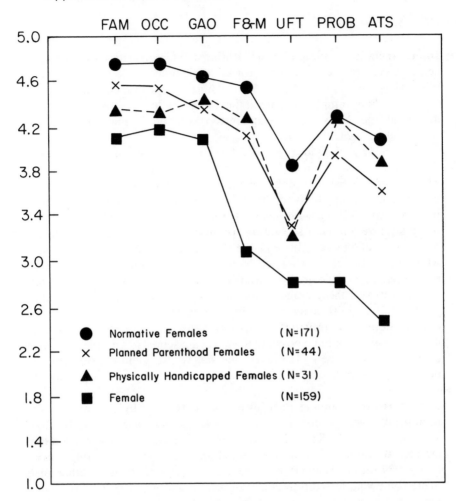

Figure 2–3. Comparison of Self-Ratings of Normative, Planned Parenthood, Physically Handicapped Females, and Outpatient Females

nonpatient samples of the same sex. These graphs clearly show that the
outpatient profile is very significantly different from that of any of the
nonpatient groups. The differences are particularly large on *Feelings and
Mood, Problems,* and *Attitude toward Self.* However, all patient scores
differ very significantly ($p < 0.01$) from the normative groups, while the
physically handicapped profile falls between the other two. It is evident,
then, that the PES scales are capable of making valid discriminations
among groups with regard to their emotional, interpersonal, and social
adjustment.

Correlational Studies

Intercorrelations among PES Self-Ratings: Intercorrelations among scale scores were obtained separately for the male and female normative samples. These are shown in table 2–6. Although specific correlations vary from sample to sample, in general there are only low positive correlations among all the scales. The average intercorrelation for males is 0.18, and for females, 0.21.

Scales 1, 2, 5, and 3, 4, 6, 7 form more highly correlated clusters for adult females, whereas 1, 2, 6, and 3, 4, 5, 7 cluster for adult males. This might suggest that problems for males in the nonpatient population center around occupation and home, whereas for women they more often involve getting along with others, feelings and mood, and self-esteem.

Intercorrelations of self-ratings on initial status for the 111 male and 159 female clients seen in 1977 are shown in table 2–7. They are somewhat higher than those obtained on the normative samples, as one would expect because of the greater variance among scores. (See tables 2–4 and 2–5.) However, the average correlation for males is only 0.24, while that for females is 0.30, again indicating that ratings on different scales are only moderately correlated. The correlations all tend to be positive, indicating that it would be possible to sum scale scores to provide an overall estimate of adjustment. However, the scales also yield considerable independent information.

Intercorrelations among PES Initial Status Ratings by Therapists: The initial status ratings of therapists were intercorrelated separately for male and female patients. These are also shown in table 2–7. These correlations are slightly higher than those obtained among patient self-ratings, averaging 0.27 for males and 0.36 for females. It appears, then, that therapists make somewhat less-differential judgment regarding areas of disturbance than do the patients. Also, recalling that the self-ratings of females are more highly correlated than those of males, whether rated by therapist or self-rated, one might speculate that problems affect women more globally than they do men.

Since ratings on the scales, whether made by clients or therapists, are moderately positively intercorrelated, they could be summed to yield an overall level of adjustment. Such a composite score might discriminate better among individuals since it would provide a more-continuous scale. Furthermore, it would be more generalizable over raters and occasions since random errors would tend to cancel each other. However, the summed score could mask real changes in certain areas of functioning and would be less informative clinically in comparing clients' functioning at reevaluation to that of the community at large. Furthermore, scores on

Table 2–6
Intercorrelations among Progress Evaluation Self-Ratings of Normative Adult Samples

Scale	Females (N = 171)						Males (N = 90)					
	2	3	4	5	6	7	2	3	4	5	6	7
1 Family Interaction	0.34	0.03	0.02	0.25	0.16	0.27	0.28	0.23	0.05	-0.03	0.47	0.10
2 Occupation		.02	.21	.15	.23	.19		.16	.02	.17	.19	.05
3 Getting Along with Others			.44	.18	.14	.30			.24	.21	.17	.22
4 Feelings and Mood				.02	.39	.34				.20	.27	.17
5 Use of Free Time					.14	.18					.20	.33
6 Problems						.49						.29
7 Attitude toward Self												

Table 2-7
Intercorrelations among Initial-Status Ratings of Patients and Therapists for Male and Female Outpatients

Scale	Males (N = 111)						Females (N = 159)					
	1	2	3	4	5	6	1	2	3	4	5	6
Patient ratings												
1 Family Interaction												
2 Occupation	21						24					
3 Getting Along with Others	05	-07					38	15				
4 Feelings and Mood	23	25	26				26	23	45			
5 Use of Free Time	19	-03	32	44			16	30	27	31		
6 Problems	11	26	24	48	35		24	17	25	53	33	
7 Attitude to Self	21	10	20	52	44	20	22	21	33	47	33	43
Therapist ratings												
1 Family Interaction												
2 Occupation	35						38					
3 Getting Along with Others	06	05					44	42				
4 Feelings and Mood	16	26	34				16	38	45			
5 Use of Free Time	13	22	25	60			21	39	45	38		
6 Problems	26	30	19	54	51		23	20	28	52	40	
7 Attitude to Self	05	08	26	40	35	24	10	38	33	53	39	50

Note: Decimal points are omitted for correlations

separate areas are of more value in answering such clinical questions as, "Could this person profit from further therapy and, if so, by what modalities and with what goals?" We expect to continue to explore how decisions can best be made regarding therapeutic efficacy with the aid of these scales, using both the separate scores and a total score.

Correlations between Initial Status Ratings of Patient and Therapist: The correlations between the initial-status scores of patient and therapist are displayed in table 2–8, with therapist ratings across and client ratings down. The italicized values are the correlations between patients and therapists for the same scale; they are all highly significant ($p < 0.01$), averaging 0.48 for females and 0.48 for males. In both samples the lowest relationships between therapists and patients are for *Family Interaction* and *Problems;* the highest are for *Occupation, Use of Free Time,* and *Attitude toward Self.* All off-diagonal correlations are lower than those on the diagonal. These correlations yield convincing evidence for the convergent and discriminant validity of the seven PES scales (Campbell and Fiske, 1959).

Intercorrelations between Patient and Therapist Goal Ratings: The means, standard deviations, and intercorrelations of patient and therapist initial-goal ratings are shown in table 2–9. Correlations between goal ratings of patient and therapist are shown in Table 2–10. These intercorrelations are much higher than were found for initial-status ratings. They average 0.53 and 0.47 for therapists rating females and males, respectively. For patients, the corresponding averages are 0.47 and 0.34.

The correlations between goals set by therapist and patient on corresponding scales are all highly significant for females. However, for males, two of the correlations—those for *Feelings and Mood,* and *Problems*—are not significantly different from zero. Furthermore, several of the off-diagonal correlations are higher than correlations on the diagonal for both males and females. Thus, the evidence is not as good for convergent and discriminant validity for goal ratings as it is for rating of current status. However, it is important to remember that goal scores for outpatients have a very limited range. Thus, low convergence and discrimination imply not that there are large differences in goals set for an individual and his or her own goals but rather that there are little individual differences in goal setting.

Correlations between Initial Status and Goal Ratings: The correlations between initial status and goals as rated by the therapists and the patients are shown in table 2–11, separately for males and females. For every scale, the therapists' goals are more highly correlated with their ratings of initial status than are those of the patients. This may be the result of

Table 2–8
Correlations between Initial Status Ratings of Patients and Therapists for Male and Female Outpatients

| | | | | | | | | *Therapist Ratings* | | | | | | |
| | Males (N = 111) | | | | | | | Females (N = 159) | | | | | | |
Scale	1	2	3	4	5	6	7	1	2	3	4	5	6	7
1 Family Interaction	*32*	15	-07	13	12	02	08	*30*	22	17	12	15	07	09
2 Occupation	32	*72*	-16	12	13	23	12	23	*62*	24	24	34	12	21
3 Getting Along with Others	09	05	*39*	19	20	01	23	17	21	*51*	21	32	22	23
4 Feelings and Mood	00	20	-09	*48*	26	31	32	-10	23	29	*40*	33	23	30
5 Use of Free Time	-06	00	06	42	*57*	13	21	05	32	26	23	*63*	25	26
6 Problems	08	16	-15	24	26	*38*	07	-01	18	22	35	22	*36*	33
7 Attitude toward Self	02	05	-02	33	26	10	*53*	06	28	25	26	23	24	*53*

Note: Decimal points are omitted for correlations. Italicized values are the correlations between patients and therapists for the same scale.

Table 2–9
Means, Standard Deviations, and Intercorrelations among Goal Ratings of Therapists and Patients

Scale	Males (N = 111)								Females (N = 159)							
	X̄	sd	1	2	3	4	5	6	X̄	sd	1	2	3	4	5	6
Patients' goal ratings																
1 Family Interaction	4.65	0.70							4.72	0.62						
2 Occupation	4.79	.49	45						4.79	.49	22					
3 Getting Along with Others	4.54	.63	21	31					4.64	.54	26	56				
4 Feelings and Mood	4.61	.64	22	33	35				4.58	.79	44	46	51			
5 Use of Free Time	4.35	.95	16	32	32	48			4.27	.99	28	45	37	61		
6 Problems	4.34	.72	13	26	29	45	39		4.39	.83	34	43	50	74	52	
7 Attitude to Self	4.32	.82	16	39	33	52	54	58	4.13	.94	19	44	50	69	57	71
Therapists' goal ratings																
1 Family Interaction	4.45	.70							4.62	.59						
2 Occupation	4.51	.83	49						4.67	.56	58					
3 Getting Along with Others	4.21	.69	28	32					4.28	.72	55	61				
4 Feelings and Mood	4.11	.79	37	40	49				4.11	.74	38	57	64			
5 Use of Free Time	3.66	.93	30	35	59	61			3.68	.92	32	52	55	63		
6 Problems	3.72	.73	33	42	50	64	61		3.72	.71	31	47	55	61	56	
7 Attitude to Self	3.82	.86	35	35	64	61	65	63	3.70	.80	35	47	58	66	57	65

Note: Decimal points are omitted for intercorrelations.

Table 2-10
Correlations between Goal Ratings of Therapists and Patients

| | Therapist Ratings | | | | | | | | | | | | |
| | Males (N = 111) | | | | | | | Females (N = 159) | | | | | | |
Scale	1	2	3	4	5	6	7	1	2	3	4	5	6	7
1 Family Interaction	44	23	00	−03	−06	−03	−04	27	29	19	17	14	09	09
2 Occupation	11	31	13	06	−03	09	05	31	52	31	35	33	24	27
3 Getting Along with Others	−01	12	33	17	17	13	10	26	43	43	26	32	33	30
4 Feelings and Mood	−08	−13	00	14	−02	−02	07	13	39	29	33	32	31	39
5 Use of Free Time	05	−03	23	34	34	18	21	08	22	20	25	34	26	29
6 Problems	−18	−08	04	13	06	06	07	12	34	23	21	16	37	33
7 Attitude toward Self	−13	04	26	31	18	21	28	10	26	24	27	27	34	38

Note: Decimal points are omitted from correlations.

Table 2–11
Correlations between PES Initial-Status and Goal Ratings for Adult Male (N = 111) and Female (N = 159) Outpatients

Scale	Therapist		Patient	
	Female	Male	Female	Male
Family Interaction	0.61	0.56	0.31	0.29
Occupation	.66	.58	.46	.26
Getting Along with Others	.76	.64	.52	.44
Feelings and Mood	.57	.40	.34	.21
Use of Free Time	.70	.42	.50	.24
Problems	.55	.44	.33	.29
Attitude toward Self	.57	.47	.32	.22

therapists' basing their goal ratings on their judgment of the patients' current functioning, history of psychopathology, motivation for change, and the like, whereas the patients probably use other information, including, possibly, their hopes and wishes for change. Also interesting is the fact that goals for females are more highly related to initial status than are those for males, whether the ratings are made by the therapist or the patient.

Relationship of PES Scores to Demographic Variables and Diagnostic Groups

Relationship to Sex, Age, Education, Marital Status, and Family Income: Present status and goal ratings of therapist and patient were analyzed for a group of 50 male and 50 female adult outpatients to determine differences in ratings as a function of sex, age, education, marital status, or income. Only the first six scales were available for analysis. There were relatively few significant relations noted except for sex. Females saw themselves as higher in *Getting Along with Others* ($p \leq 0.01$) and lower in *Feelings and Mood* ($p \leq 0.05$) than did males. However, this difference did not hold for a new sample. The therapists also rated the women higher on *Getting Along with Others* and somewhat but not significantly lower in mood than they did the men. Female patients rated their goals higher for occupation and peer relations than did male patients (table 2–12).

Relatively few correlations between demographic variables and ratings were significant at the 0.05 level, and those that were tended to occur with ratings of males. In particular, the therapists' ratings of occupational status were higher for males who were older, better educated, in higher-income brackets, and married, but these relations did not hold for ratings of females. Married men saw themselves as having better family interactions and set higher goals on this dimension than did single

Table 2–12
Correlations of PES with Demographic Variables

Scale		Males (N = 50)		Correlations				Females (N = 50)		Correlations			
		Mean	sd	Age	Educa-tion	Marital Status	Income	Mean	sd	Age	Educa-tion	Marital Status	Income
Present family interaction	Patient	3.94	0.84	0.12	-0.18	0.34*	0.20	3.94	0.89	-0.13	0.13	0.09	0.33*
	Therapist	3.84	.65	.14	-.05	.07	.16	4.00	.61	.11	.00	-.14	.06
Goals family interaction	Patient	4.76	.52	.03	-.03	.43**	.12	4.84	.42	-.13	.08	.07	.16
	Therapist	4.46	.54	.04	.01	.00	.05	4.48	.61	-.09	.00	.15	.03
Present occupation	Patient	4.06	1.17	.41**	.08	.23	.42**	3.88	1.12	-.01	.03	.07	.19
	Therapist	3.92	1.28	.35**	.45**	.32*	.57**	3.92	1.01	-.04	.06	.15	.11
Goals occupation	Patient	4.80*	.45	-.12	-.03	.14	.12	4.96*	.20	-.26	-.26	.07	-.01
n	Therapist	3.54	.61	.12	.09	.23	.52**	4.60	.57	-.17	-.10	.16	.07
Present getting along	Patient	3.70**	.86	.19	-.01	.22	.03	4.14**	.83	.14	.22	-.03	.15
	Therapist	3.34*	.92	-.04	.06	.37*	.02	3.76*	.77	.22	.18	-.12	-.04
Goals getting along	Patient	4.46*	.58	.03	-.15	-.08	-.20	4.68*	.51	.03	.17	-.12	.07
	Therapist	4.04	.67	-.07	-.01	.24	.06	4.22	.58	.16	.04	-.09	-.06
Present feelings and mood	Patient	3.46*	1.15	-.03	-.09	-.04	-.08	2.94*	1.18	.20	.16	.14	.19
	Therapist	2.94	1.15	-.19	.09	.09	.04	2.78	.91	.29*	.06	.01	.09

Goals feelings and mood	Patient	4.50	.79	−.12	.05	.09	.10	4.74	.56	.03	.01	.04	.23
	Therapist	4.10	.76	−.26	−.02	−.04	.01	4.10	.68	.17	−.08	.11	.07
Present use of free time	Patient	3.02	1.25	−.07	.04	.01	−.21	2.96	1.34	.20	.26	.07	.13
	Therapist	2.78	1.13	.11	.12	.13	.05	2.98	.87	.09	.12	−.06	.03
Goals use of free time	Patient	4.38	.80	.00	.05	.05	.00	4.48	.89	.06	.08	.06	.06
	Therapist	3.84	.74	.04	−.01	.24	.17	4.04	.67	.05	−.00	−.15	−.09
Present problems	Patient	2.84	1.09	−.13	.19	.16	.01	2.72	1.03	.08	.01	.22	.26
	Therapist	2.80	.99	−.05	.21	−.03	−.05	2.74	.80	−.01	−.06	−.02	−.03
Goals problems	Patient	4.42	.78	−.33*	.02	.03	.01	4.42	.73	−.04	−.16	.12	.15
	Therapist	3.94	.65	−.14	.10	.02	−.04	3.92	.63	.03	−.16	−.09	−.10

*p < 0.05.
**p < 0.01.

Table 2–13
Profiles of Initial Status of Various Diagnostic Groups

							Therapist Ratings						
Diagnostic Group	*Family Interaction*		Occupation		Getting Along with Others		Feelings and Mood		Use of Free Time		Problems	
	X̄	sd	X̄	sd	X̄	sd	X̄	sd	X̄	sd	X̄	sd
Organic brain syndrome	2.67	1.23	2.80	1.21	2.80	0.56	2.33	1.05	2.47	1.25	2.33	0.82
Psychoses	3.24	.92	3.08	1.32	3.24	1.05	3.20	1.22	2.60	1.12	2.44	.77
Personality disorder,	3.68	.85	3.92	1.00	3.28	.94	2.84	1.07	2.56	1.26	3.04	.73
Neuroses	4.24	.78	4.00	.82	3.76	.72	2.48	.87	2.80	1.12	3.12	.60
Adjustment reaction	4.00	.58	4.04	1.10	4.16	.69	3.16	.94	2.96	1.17	3.16	.80
					Patient Ratings							
Personality disorder	3.56	.82	3.44	1.32	3.52	1.19	2.64	1.47	2.20	1.12	3.28	.74
Neuroses	3.96	1.14	4.00	1.00	3.84	1.11	3.00	1.32	3.28	1.21	3.20	.82
Adjustment reaction	4.08	.64	4.04	1.14	4.32	.75	3.32	1.34	3.16	1.52	3.20	.71

Note: All diagnostic groups consisted of 25 patients with the exception of organic brain syndrome, for which $N = 15$.

men. In both samples that were analyzed, older males set lower goals for relief of problems than did younger men. For females, higher income was correlated with better family interaction.

In summary, our studies to date indicate that demographic variables such as age, sex, marital status, income, and education have very few, if any, consistent effects on status ratings of therapists and patients on all scales with the possible exception of *Family Interaction* and *Occupation*.

Comparison among Diagnostic Groups: Comparisons were made among four diagnostic groups on the basis of therapists' ratings of initial status. The four diagnostic categories were: neuroses, psychoses, personality disorder, and adjustment reaction. For each category, 25 successive patients with appropriate diagnosis were drawn. The first six scales were used to compare the groups; the seventh, *Attitude toward Self,* had not yet been developed. The means and standard deviations of ratings of opening status are displayed in table 2–13. A fifth diagnostic group—organic brain syndrome—is also shown. Only 15 patients comprised this group.

Multivariate analyses of variance were carried out comparing neurotics with psychotics and personality disorders with adjustment reactions. The results are shown in table 2–14. Both analyses revealed highly significant overall differences ($p < 0.00001$ and $p < 0.001$, respectively), indicating that the corresponding profiles are essentially different.

Turning now to the comparisons for individual scales, we note that

Table 2–14
Multivariate Analysis of Diagnostic Groupings

Scale	F	df	p
Comparison: Neuroses versus Psychoses			
Overall	9.15	6,43	0.00001
Family Interaction	17.08	1,48	.001
Occupation	8.78	1,48	.005
Getting Along with Others	4.15	1,48	.05
Feelings and Mood	5.73	1,48	.05
Use of Free Time	.40	1,48	ns
Problems	27.16	1,48	.001
Comparison: Personality Disorder versus Adjustment Reaction			
Overall	5.03	6,43	.001
Family Interaction	2.42	1,48	ns
Occupation	.16	1,48	ns
Getting Along with Others	29.16	1,48	.001
Feelings and Mood	1.26	1,48	ns
Use of Free Time	1.35	1,48	ns
Problems	.31	1,48	ns

five of the six scales differentiated neurotics and psychotics. Neurotics were rated significantly higher than psychotics on *Family Interaction, Occupation, Getting Along with Others,* and *Problems.* They were significantly lower on *Feelings and Mood* (figures 2–4 and 2–5).

Although in general, patients diagnosed as having adjustment reactions were rated higher than those diagnosed as personality disorder, only one scale, taken by itself, revealed a significant difference: *Getting Along with Others.* This scale tends to differentiate personality disorder, ad-

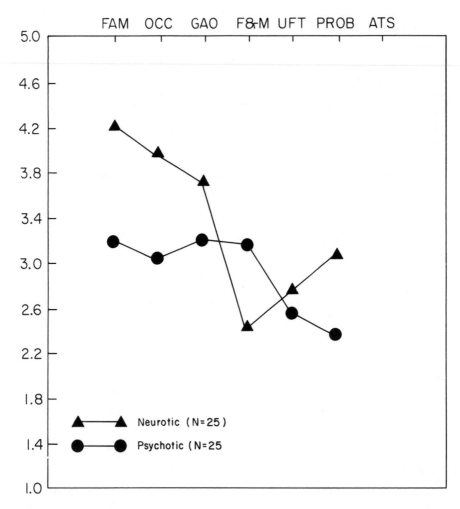

Figure 2–4. Comparison of Neurotic to Psychotic Outpatients: Ratings by Therapists

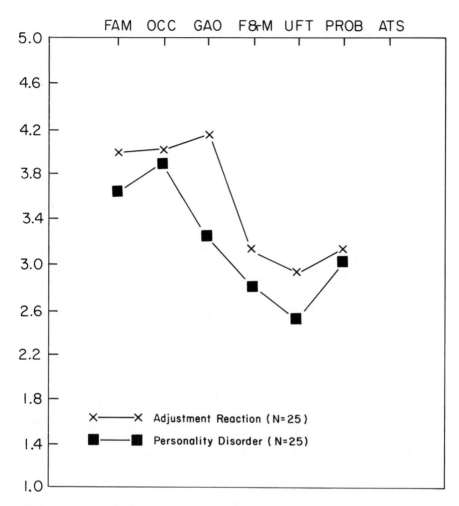

Figure 2–5. Comparison of Personality Disorders to Adjustment-Reaction Outpatients: Ratings by Therapists

justment reactions, and neurotics, the scores for the last diagnosis falling about midway between those of the other two. *Feelings and Mood* also differentiates the three groups but not to the same extent; here the neurotics are lowest.

Table 2–13 also presents the average scores on present status as rated by the patient for all but the psychotic patients and organic brain syndrome. What is most interesting about these scores are the ways in which they differ from the therapists' ratings. The neurotic patients see themselves as having less disturbance in *Feelings and Mood* and in *Use of Free Time* than indicated by the therapists. The latter difference is significant (p <0.05). Patients diagnosed as personality disorder, on the other hand, tend to rate themselves as more disturbed (lower) on both these scales, but rate themselves very significantly lower on *Occupation*. Overall patients in these latter two diagnostic categories appear to differ more from the therapist in their ratings than do patients with adjustment reactions.

Due to the possibility of sex differences and in order to obtain information on the seventh scale *(Attitude toward Self)*, later data were obtained and analyzed among diagnostic groups comparing males and females separately on initial-status ratings of the PES scales (table 2–15). This analysis reveals significant differences among diagnostic groups on five of the seven scales for females, but only on *Getting Along with Others* for males, based on therapists' ratings. Examining the profiles of these groups (figures 2–6 and 2–7), we note that for females, adjustment-reaction and personality-disorder groups have almost parallel profiles, but the adjustment-reaction group is significantly higher on *Family Interaction, Occupation, Getting Along with Others,* and *Attitude toward Self*. The adjustment-reaction group is significantly higher than neurotics on *Getting Along with Others* and on *Feelings and Mood*. While trends are similar for therapists' ratings of male patients, the groups differ significantly only for *Getting Along with Others*, with adjustment reaction scoring higher than neurotics and both scoring higher than personality disorders.

These results are consistent with our previous findings based on a mixed sample of males and females and further indicate that differences among these diagnostic groups on the PES scales are primarily attributable to females.

Self-ratings were available for the more-recent (1977) data and provided interesting additional findings (table 2–15). Males diagnosed as personality disorders rated themselves higher relative to therapists on all but one scale, *Family Interaction*, with almost all the mean differences significant. They also rated themselves significantly higher than either of the other diagnostic groups on *Feelings and Mood, Use of Free Time,* and *Problem* severity. There were no differences among the self-ratings of female diagnostic groups, but those diagnosed personality disorder also tended to rate themselves higher than did their therapists on several of the scales, with the difference on *Getting Along with Others* and *Problems* reaching significance (p <0.05).

For the more-recent sample, initial-goal ratings made by the therapists and patients were also analyzed to determine if they varied with diagnostic grouping. The mean goal ratings are shown in table 2–16 for males and

Table 2–15
Mean Ratings of PES Initial Status for Various Outpatient Diagnostic Groups

Scale	Neurosis[a] Therapist	Patient	Adjustment Reaction[b] Therapist	Patient	Personality Disorder[c] Therapist	Patient[e]	Other[d] Therapist	Patient	Combined Within-Group sd Therapist	Patient	Probability of No Difference among Groups Therapist	Patient
Females												
Family Interaction	4.13	4.09	4.12	4.15	3.74	3.97	4.20	4.20	0.64	0.72	0.01	
Occupation	4.11	4.20	4.24	4.15	3.94	4.17	4.70	4.35	.86	.85	.01	
Getting Along with Others	3.51	4.20	3.97	4.09	3.38	3.81	4.45	4.25	.90	.91	.001	
Feelings and Mood	2.60	2.89	3.04	3.19	2.81	3.00	3.20	3.25	.92	1.20	.04	
Use of Free Time	2.69	2.78	2.82	2.84	2.51	2.92	2.95	2.75	1.14	1.53		
Problems	2.62	2.78	2.65	2.82	2.38	2.89	2.85	2.95	.86	1.06		
Attitude toward Self	2.49	2.31	2.61	2.56	2.16	2.47	2.95	2.58	.92	1.03	.05	
Males												
Family Interaction	4.08	3.96	3.80	3.86	3.77	3.73	3.71	3.79	.62	.89		
Occupation	3.64	4.04	3.59	3.69	3.82	4.45	3.79	4.36	1.41	1.27		.085
Getting Along with Others	3.44	3.84	4.04	4.08	2.95	4.41	3.36	4.00	.93	.91	.001	
Feelings and Mood	2.68	2.88	2.80	2.94	2.64	3.82	3.00	3.57	1.08	1.24		.02
Use of Free Time	2.48	2.68	2.65	2.51	2.64	3.41	2.50	2.43	1.10	1.33		.05
Problems	2.52	2.64	2.59	2.39	2.59	3.41	2.57	3.00	.98	1.14		.01
Attitude toward Self	2.17	2.54	2.79	2.71	2.67	3.06	2.50	2.67	.99	1.15		.09

[a] N = 45 for females and N = 25 for males.
[b] N = 74 for females and N = 49 for males.
[c] N = 47 for females and N = 22 for males.
[d] N = 20 for females and N = 14 for males.
[e] N = 36.

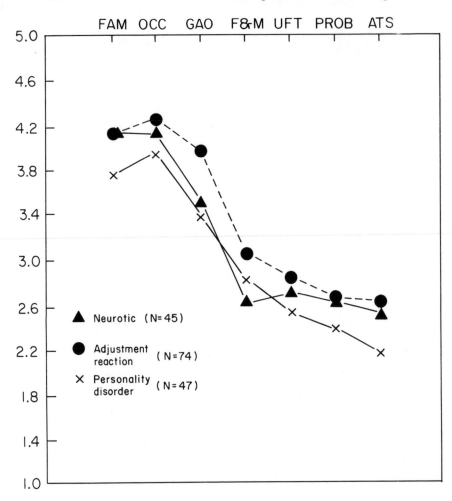

Figure 2–6. Comparison of Neurotic, Adjustment-Reaction, and Personality-Disorder Female Outpatients: Ratings by Therapists

females separately. The miscellaneous diagnostic grouping "other" has been omitted.

Overall significantly different goals are set for a number of scales for the various diagnostic groups as rated by patients and therapists for the male sample, and by therapists for the female sample. Furthermore, for both sets of ratings, the highest goals on most scales are set by therapists for men diagnosed as adjustment reactions. However, the patients diagnosed personality disorders set nearly as high goals as did those termed adjustment reaction. It is the neurotic group who set the lowest goals,

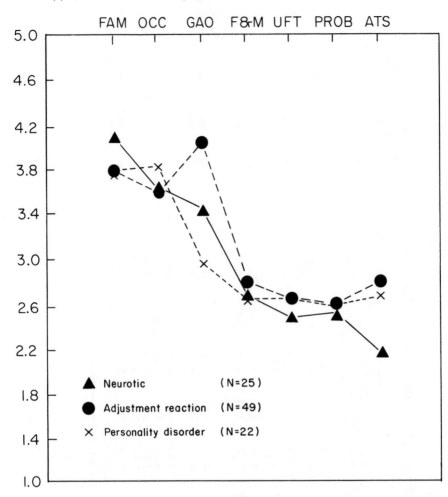

Figure 2–7. Comparison of Neurotic, Adjustment-Reaction, and Personality-Disorder Male Outpatients: Ratings by Therapists

significantly lower than the adjustment-reaction group on five of the seven scales. The therapists also set goals on the *Feelings and Mood* and *Attitude toward Self* scales significantly lower for neurotics as compared to the group diagnosed adjustment reactions. But they also set lower goals on these two scales plus *Getting Along with Others* and *Use of Free Time* for personality disorders compared to adjustment reactions.

The therapists set significantly lower goals on every scale for females diagnosed personality disorder as compared to adjustment reaction. They also set significantly lower goals for them as compared to neurotics on all but *Feeling and Mood* and *Occupation*. Goals on *Feelings and Mood*,

Table 2–16
Mean Initial Goal Ratings by Therapists and Patients for Groups Classified by Sex and Diagnostic Group

Scale	Neurosis[a]		Problem of Adjustment[b]		Personality Disorder[c]		Combined Within-Group sd		Probability of No Difference among Groups	
	Therapist	Patient	Therapist	Patient	Therapist	Patient[d]	Therapist	Patient	Therapist	Patient
Females										
Family Interaction	4.69	4.69	4.70	4.74	4.17**	4.83	0.57	0.62	0.002	ns
Occupation	4.60	4.87	4.77	4.74	4.28*	4.83	.54	.49	.002	ns
Getting Along with Others	4.18*	4.69	4.44	4.66	3.68**	4.47	.68	.55	.000	ns
Feelings and Mood	3.78*	4.42	4.35	4.69	3.64*	4.72	.70	.78	.000	ns
Use of Free Time	3.53*	4.27	3.90	4.30	3.07**	4.25	.90	.99	.01	ns
Problems	3.64	4.34	3.89	4.51	3.11**	4.33	.69	.83	.002	ns
Attitude toward Self	3.56*	4.14	3.92	4.28	3.07**	4.11	.77	.93	.002	ns
Males										
Family Interaction	4.56	4.44	4.51	4.76	4.23	4.68	0.70	0.70	ns	ns
Occupation	4.64	4.52	4.59	4.88	4.23	4.77	.83	.47	ns	.01
Getting Along with Others	4.16	4.40	4.49	4.65	3.86*	4.54	.64	.63	.001	ns
Feelings and Mood	3.88*	4.32	4.35	4.69	3.82*	4.54	.77	.62	.02	.02
Use of Free Time	3.56	3.92	3.94	4.55	3.32*	4.18	.91	.92	.03	.02
Problems	3.64	3.80	3.86	4.59	3.54	4.23	.73	.65	ns	.02
Attitude toward Self	3.62*	3.83	4.17	4.62	3.44*	4.06	.81	.76	.001	.001

*Significantly different from mean for adjustment reaction.
**Significantly different from mean for adjustment reaction and neurosis.
[a]N = 45 for females and N = 25 for males.
[b]N = 74 for females and N = 49 for males.
[c]N = 47 for females and N = 22 for males.
[d]N = 36.

Use of Free Time, and *Attitude toward Self* are all set lower for neurotic patients as compared to adjustment reactions.

Inpatients versus Outpatients: One additional comparison that has been analyzed is that between 25 sequentially drawn adult inpatients from Ypsilanti State Hospital and 25 outpatients from Shiawassee Mental Health Center. For this comparison, both present status and goals were examined using therapists' ratings. The results are illustrated in figure 2–8.

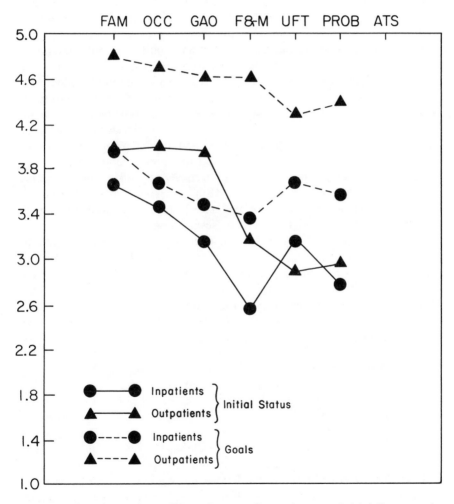

Figure 2–8. Comparison of Inpatients to Outpatients on Initial Status and Goals: Ratings by Therapists

The two groups differed significantly in present functioning by a multivariate F test. Two scales yielded significant differences—*Getting Along with Others* and *Feelings and Mood*—with inpatients rated lower. However, the most striking difference found was for goals. As clearly seen in figure 2–8, the goals for each scale were set very significantly lower for inpatients than for outpatients.

Sensitivity of PES to Therapeutic Intervention

Evaluation at Termination: In an early study utilizing the first six scales, termination data were analyzed on 69 clients. For 25 clients, final evaluations were obtained from both the patient and the therapist; for the remaining 44, final evaluations were obtained only from the therapist.

For the first analysis, all 69 cases were used, and means, standard deviations, and intercorrelations were obtained among initial evaluations, goals, and therapists' ratings of outcome. For the 25 cases with client-outcome evaluations, an additional analysis was run including client-outcome evaluations. The age, education, and diagnosis of the client, the therapy, the number of therapy sessions, and time elapsing from opening to closing of the case were also included in the correlation matrix.

The total sample consisted of 42 females and 27 males averaging 32.5 years of age and ranging from 18 to 50. Two-thirds of the clients had a high-school education or better, 31 were diagnosed adjustment reactions, and the average number of sessions was 4.4, sd 2.64, over an average interval of 2.4 ± 1.6 months. The means and standard deviations of scores on the evaluation scales are given in table 2–17. A comparison of the opening and termination scores reveals that the patients improved, on the average, on all scales, but the changes were minimal for *Family Interaction, Occupation,* and *Getting Along with Others.* Much more sizable changes were indicated for *Feelings and Mood, Use of Free Time,* and *Problems,* as illustrated in figure 2–9. These were also the areas that both the patient and the therapist considered to be most impaired at the beginning of treatment.

The subsample of 25 patients who also evaluated themselves at closing consisted of 18 females and 7 males and averaged 5.2 therapy sessions over two to seven months. Their opening evaluations are very similar to those of the total group except that they are somewhat more homogeneous (smaller standard deviations on many scales). They were rated higher at closing by the therapists than was the total group.

What is most striking in table 2–18 is the extent to which the patients' closing evaluations exceed those of the therapists. The difference ranges from 0.12 for *Occupation* to 0.60 for *Use of Free Time.* For only one

Table 2-17
Means and Standard Deviations of Scores on Evaluation Scales for Sixty-nine Patients Evaluated at Beginning and Termination of Therapy

	Family Interaction		Occupation		Getting Along with Others		Feelings and Mood		Use of Free Time		Problems	
	X	sd	X	sd	X	sd	X	sd	X	sd	X	sd
Opening												
Therapist	3.88	0.78	4.09	1.11	3.74	0.87	3.06	1.03	2.74	1.13	2.88	0.91
Patient	3.97	.73	4.13	1.10	3.99	.96	3.23	1.27	3.26	1.36	2.83	1.12
Goals												
Therapist	4.72	.48	4.74	.47	4.46	.58	4.46	.56	4.17	.77	4.29	.67
Patient	4.88	.32	4.90	.41	4.78	.42	4.86	.35	4.75	.58	4.66	.47
Termination												
Therapist	4.03	.69	4.14	.99	3.96	.78	3.64	.77	3.48	1.05	3.46	.83

Table 2-18
Means and Standard Deviations of Scores on Evaluation Scales for Twenty-five Patients Evaluated at Beginning and Termination of Therapy by Therapist and Patient

	Family Interaction		Occupation		Getting Along with Others		Feelings and Mood		Use of Free Time		Problems	
	X	sd	X	sd	X	sd	X	sd	X	sd	X	sd
Opening												
Therapist	4.08	0.57	4.24	0.88	3.80	0.96	3.04	0.98	2.68	1.11	3.12	0.67
Patient	4.04	.45	4.36	.99	4.20	.87	3.20	1.19	3.36	1.35	2.84	1.21
Goals												
Therapist	4.80	.41	4.76	.44	4.56	.51	4.44	.51	4.28	.61	4.44	.51
Patient	4.96	.20	5.00	.00	4.76	.44	4.84	.37	4.64	.76	4.76	.44
Termination												
Therapist	4.28	.54	4.44	.77	4.12	.73	3.76	.66	3.60	1.04	3.60	.76
Patient	4.76	.44	4.56	1.00	4.44	.71	4.32	.99	4.20	1.08	4.12	1.09

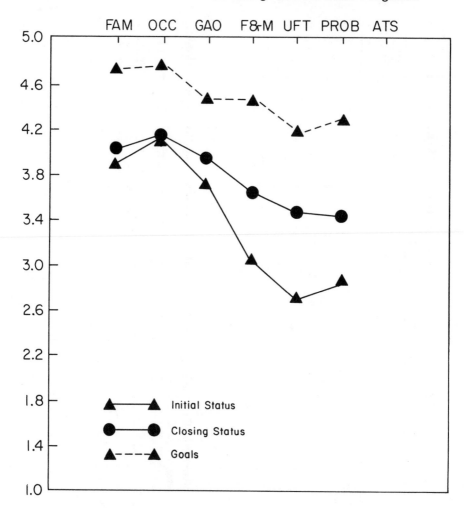

Figure 2–9. Comparison of Initial Status, Goals, and Closing Status for Mixed Group of Male and Female Outpatients (N = 69): Ratings by Therapists

variable—*Use of Free Time*—was there a large difference in rating to begin with. Neither set of closing evaluations was as high as the initial goals.

Correlations between sex, age, education, diagnosis, number of sessions, and elapsed time since intake and each of the outcome ratings were computed. Although levels of significance are reported here, it should be noted that they may be misleading since the distribution of scores at closing tends to be skewed. The values obtained were, for the most part, low and inconsistent (table 2-19). Those found with sex and education were similar to trends noted previously with some intake data; females were higher than males on *Family Interaction* (p <0.01) and *Getting Along with Others* (p ≤0.05), and education was positively correlated with *Occupation* (p <0.05). Another interesting relationship found was that the diagnosis of adjustment reaction was positively related with closing status on *Feelings and Mood* and on *Problems,* according to the therapist ($r = 0.28$ and $r = 0.27$, p <0.05). Length of time in treatment was positively correlated with all ratings, but the correlations for the most part were quite small, and only that for therapist rating of *Family Interaction* reached significance (p <0.05).

Another set of correlations of interest are those between the initial ratings of therapist and patient and the therapists' final ratings. These are shown in table 2-20. An interesting pattern becomes evident. Therapists' final ratings are highly correlated with their ratings of initial status on the first three scales but not on the last three. We had already noted a relationship between demographic variables and two of the first three scales. Thus, one suspects that these scales tap more-enduring aspects of the patient's life, perhaps dependent upon the overall life-style and on socioeconomic factors. The scales dealing with moods, use of free time, and severity of problems, on the other hand, appear to measure more-temporary aspects that are not deeply rooted and are more amenable to modification. It is of interest to note that for these scales, outcome is more highly related to goals than to initial status, whereas the opposite is true for the first three.

There is little relationship between patient's opening rating and the therapist's closing except for the first two scales.

A more-recent study of termination outcome was carried out on a sample of 44 males and 58 females who filled out and returned the consumer satisfaction questionnaire and PES ratings within three months after termination of therapy. They were matched by sex, age, and diagnosis to 42 males and 58 females seen during the same period of time who did not return the questionnaire. The means and standard deviations of their PES ratings and those of their therapists for initial status, goals, and closing status are shown in tables 2-21, 2-22, 2-23 and 2-24.

These data were analyzed in a number of ways. The first question was whether there was a difference on any of the PES ratings of initial status between those who returned the questionnaires and those who did not was examined. Data in tables 2-21 and 2-23 were compared, as were those in table 2-22 and 2-24. It was noted that opening-status scores were higher for those returning the questionnaires than for their matched controls, whether rated by therapist or patient, but the differences

Table 2–19

Correlations between Outcome Measures and Demographic and Treatment Variables

	Outcome								
	Family Interaction			Occupation			Getting Along with Others		
	Therapist		Patient	Therapist		Patient	Therapist		Patient
Variable	(N=69)	(N=25)	(N=25)	(N=69)	(N=25)	(N=25)	(N=69)	(N=25)	(N=25)
Sex	43**	16	07	21	−23	−10	30*	11	52*
Age	−03	−07	−29	09	20	05	02	06	−31
Education	17	23	06	19	22	44*	17	−02	−29
Diagnosis (Adjustment reaction versus "other")	09	−36	−21	−04	−35	−06	13	−05	31
Number of sessions	12	36	−06	03	34	30	09	17	−21
Time in treatment	25*	30	20	12	38	28	11	14	23

Note: Decimal points are omitted from correlations.

*$p \leq 0.05$.

**$p \leq 0.01$.

Table 2–20

Correlations between Initial Ratings of Patient and Therapist and Final Ratings of Therapist (N = 69)

		Therapist Closing Ratings					
		1	2	3	4	5	6
Therapist opening ratings							
1	Family Interaction: Present	64	40	31	13	21	40
	Family Interaction: Goals	43	09	28	20	26	18
2	Occupation: Present	36	73	26	19	15	13
	Occupation: Goals	16	40	29	22	28	27
3	Getting Along with Others: Present	31	23	44	21	17	23
	Getting Along with Others: Goals	37	16	37	38	38	34
4	Feelings and Mood: Present	23	39	28	21	29	29
	Feelings and Mood: Goals	20	−02	29	23	27	23
5	Use of Free Time: Present	02	20	19	19	25	19
	Use of Free Time: Goals	27	14	24	31	37	29
6	Problems: Present	24	18	26	09	24	24
	Problems: Goals	34	25	39	32	43	44
Patient opening ratings							
1	Family Interaction: Present	33	25	10	01	15	22
	Family Interaction: Goals	28	28	16	18	25	20
2	Occupation: Present	35	63	30	30	21	21
	Occupation: Goals	29	40	19	15	19	24
3	Getting Along with Others: Present	31	20	18	03	17	19
	Getting Along with Others: Goals	−08	−10	−12	−20	07	00
4	Feelings and Mood: Present	09	25	14	24	04	12
	Feelings and Mood: Goals	02	27	19	07	23	03
5	Use of Free Time: Present	04	−03	02	−11	10	09
	Use of Free Time: Goals	−09	−04	−06	−01	20	12
6	Problems: Present	−11	18	−03	−11	−15	−16
	Problems: Goals	−15	01	−04	03	−09	−12

Note: Decimal points are omitted from correlations.

Outcome								
Feelings and Mood			Use of Free Time			Problems		
Therapist		Patient	Therapist		Patient	Therapist		Patient
(N=69)	(N=25)	(N=25)	(N=69)	(N=25)	(N=25)	(N=69)	(N=25)	(N=25)
09	04	30	.−09	−16	12	02	−21	07
−11	−07	21	02	27	−18	−09	14	−12
14	−10	−39	29*	21	05	25*	10	−10
28*	−14	−07	20	14	−11	27*	19	−41*
02	09	−14	15	29	04	07	28	24
13	26	21	17	20	29	13	17	32

reached significance on only two ratings for the females and two for the males, all made by the therapists. Only one of the differences in patient self-ratings reached significance. The females returning the questionnaire made better *Use of Free Time* (p <0.001) and had somewhat less-severe *Problems* (p <0.005) according to the therapist than did the controls. For the males, the significant differences were for *Family Interaction* (p <0.01) and *Feelings and Mood* (p <0.01). Goals were almost identical for the two groups, and relatively few differences were noted on closing status. One other piece of information that did differentiate the two groups, however, was number of therapy sessions. Females returning the questionnaire had an average of 10.9 sessions, and males 11.0 sessions compared to 6.4 and 8.2 sessions, respectively, for those not returning the material. This finding could imply that a longer, and possibly more-satisfying, relationship between therapist and patient may be what is most important in getting the patient to give feedback to the clinic. Possibly there was better communication between the two from the beginning as indicated by the fact that initial ratings of therapist and patient were somewhat closer for those returning the material than for those who did not. Of course, it is also possible that those not returning the ratings did not share their therapists' optimism as to the outcome of therapy.

Comparing therapist closing status to opening status, it is evident that, on average, all four groups made substantial gains in adjustment. The largest gains were obtained uniformly on *Feelings and Mood,* followed by *Problems* and *Attitude toward Self.* These are the areas where there is most room for improvement as judged by the initial-status profiles. The males who returned the questionnaire also showed a sizable gain in

Table 2–21
PES Means and Standard Deviations for Females Returning Consumer Satisfaction Questionnaire

Scale		Opening Status		Opening Goals		Closing Status	
		Therapist	Patient	Therapist	Patient	Therapist	Patient
Family Interaction	X̄	4.10	4.17	4.62	4.62	4.31	4.55
	sd	.61	.73	.59	.72	.65	.73
Occupation	X̄	4.26	4.26	4.60	4.79	4.47	4.66
	sd	.78	.85	.62	.49	.71	.64
Getting Along with Others	X̄	3.79	4.12	4.21	4.60	4.21	4.43
	sd	.87	.92	.67	.56	.72	.73
Feelings and Mood	X̄	2.91	3.00	4.02	4.53	3.93	4.06
	sd	.84	1.04	.69	.86	.72	1.07
Use of Free Time	X̄	3.14***	3.31*	3.81	4.55	3.62***	3.86
	sd	1.05	1.48	.93	.84	.93	1.28
Problems	X̄	2.86**	2.86	3.74	4.34	3.60**	4.03
	sd	.76	1.07	.69	.97	.90	.97
Attitude to Self	X̄	2.66	2.47	3.70	4.17	3.60*	3.50
	sd	.88	.97	.85	.99	.90	1.27

Note: Subjects matched by age, sex, and diagnosis to patients who did not return CSQ.

$***$ < .001 ⎫
$**$ < .005 ⎬ Significantly higher than clients who did not return the CSQ.
$*$ < .01 ⎭

Table 2–22
PES Means and Standard Deviations for Males Returning Consumer Satisfaction Questionnaire (N = 44)

Scale		Opening Status		Opening Goals		Closing Status	
		Therapist	Patient	Therapist	Patient	Therapist	Patient
Family Interaction	X̄	4.02*	3.95	4.57	4.59	4.20	4.39
	sd	.66	.78	.66	.84	.67	.89
Occupation	X̄	3.75	4.02	4.48	4.73	4.23*	4.36
	sd	1.40	1.23	.93	.54	.86	1.14
Getting Along with Others	X̄	3.73	4.14	4.25	4.57	4.05	4.20
	sd	.97	.93	.65	.55	.75	.93
Feelings and Mood	X̄	3.05*	3.34	4.16	4.55	3.82	3.75
	sd	.94	1.06	.71	.63	.76	1.26
Use of Free Time	X̄	2.82	2.93	3.82	4.39	3.39	3.39
	sd	1.04	1.34	.76	1.06	.99	1.28
Problems	X̄	2.80	2.93	3.77	4.30	3.52	3.52
	sd	.82	1.04	.64	.79	.98	1.23
Attitude to Self	X̄	2.72	2.78	3.83	4.31	3.43	3.45
	sd	1.06	1.04	.85	.95	1.00	1.41

Note: Subjects matched by age, sex, and diagnosis to patients who did not return the CSQ.
*$p < 0.01$. Significantly higher than clients who did not return CSQ.

Table 2–23
PES Means and Standard Deviations for Females Not Returning Consumer Satisfaction Questionnaire (N = 58)

Scale		Opening Status		Opening Goals		Closing Status
		Therapist	Patient	Therapist	Patient	Therapist
Family Interaction	X̄	3.95	4.00	4.48	4.67	4.21
	sd	.71	.80	.68	.66	.74
Occupation	X̄	4.03	4.01	4.55	4.76	4.21
	sd	1.06	.93	.60	.47	.87
Getting Along with Others	X̄	3.62	4.02	4.16	4.66	4.03
	sd	.99	.95	.77	.48	.82
Feelings and Mood	X̄	2.66	3.14	4.00	4.62	3.71
	sd	.93	1.29	.77	.67	.96
Use of Free Time	X̄	2.48***	2.76*	3.55	4.28	2.91***
	sd	1.08	1.53	.94	.93	1.03
Problems	X̄	2.43**	2.76	3.95	4.39	3.12**
	sd	.84	1.10	.75	.70	1.10
Attitude to Self	X̄	2.53	2.62	3.64	4.14	3.16*
	sd	.84	1.09	.77	.85	1.13

Note: Subjects matched by age, sex, and diagnosis to patients who returned CSQ.
*** < 0.001. Significantly lower than clients who returned CSQ.
** < 0.005. Significantly lower than clients who returned CSQ.
* < 0.01. Significantly lower than clients who returned CSQ.

Table 2–24
PES Means and Standard Deviations for Males Not Returning Consumer Satisfaction Questionnaire

Scale		Opening Status		Opening Goals		Closing Status
		Therapist	Patient	Therapist	Patient	Therapist
Family Interaction	$\overline{X}$	3.71*	3.67	4.36	4.64	4.00
	sd	.55	.93	.73	.66	.66
Occupation	$\overline{X}$	3.55	3.83	4.48	4.80	3.74*
	sd	1.38	1.38	.67	.45	1.19
Getting Along with Others	$\overline{X}$	3.60	4.10	4.19	4.50	4.00
	sd	.94	.88	.67	.71	.86
Feelings and Mood	$\overline{X}$	2.52*	2.95	4.14	4.67	3.62
	sd	1.02	1.38	.78	.65	.91
Use of Free Time	$\overline{X}$	2.45	2.52	3.62	4.38	3.02
	sd	1.09	1.37	.88	.85	.95
Problems	$\overline{X}$	2.47	2.55	3.79	4.33	3.33
	sd	.99	1.19	.65	.72	.90
Attitude to Self	$\overline{X}$	2.45	2.52	3.86	4.31	3.26
	sd	.86	1.09	.75	.86	.94

Note: Subjects matched by age, sex, and diagnosis to patients who returned CSQ.
*< 0.01. Significantly lower than clients who returned CSQ.

Occupation—significantly more than did their controls. While goals were reached, on average, for only one or two scales, results appeared reasonably satisfactory on the whole (figure 2–10).

Closing-status self-ratings were made only by those clients returning the questionnaire. These ratings are compared to their opening status and goal ratings in figures 2–11 and 2–12. These figures suggest that the

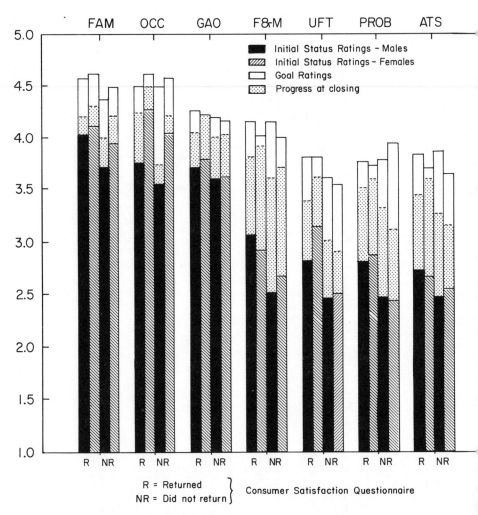

Figure 2–10. Comparison of Therapists' Ratings for Outpatients Returning and Not Returning CSQ: Groups Matched by Age and Diagnosis

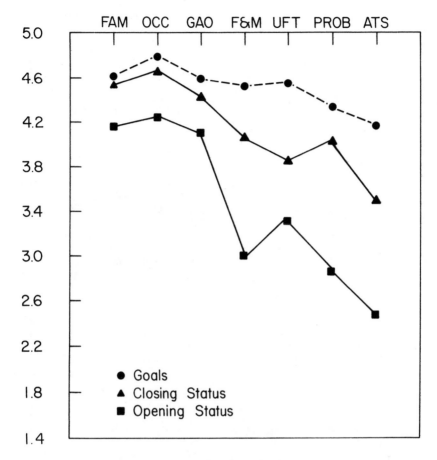

Figure 2–11. Initial Status, Goals, and Closing Status for Female Outpatients Returning CSQ: Self-Ratings (N = 58)

women considered themselves somewhat more improved than did the
men, particularly on *Feelings and Mood* and *Problems*.

   A somewhat different method of comparing outcome for patients who
returned the consumer satisfaction questionnaire with those who did not
was investigated. This method involved counting the number of times
that the therapist's closing-status ratings on each scale reached or exceeded the initial goals. The ratings for initial status, goals, and closing-
status were also summed separately to obtain total closing scores for each
person, and these scores were compared to determine the frequency with
which the overall goals were reached or exceeded. The results of this
analysis are shown in table 2–25. These data show that specific goals on

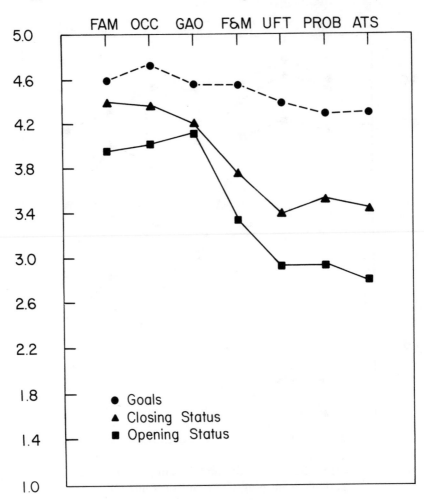

Figure 2–12. Initial Status, Goals, and Closing Status for Male Outpatients Returning CSQ: Self-Ratings (N = 44)

any one scale were reached for well over half the sample, with only four exceptions. These exceptions were for *Use of Free Time* and *Attitude toward Self* on which fewer than half of both males and females not returning the questionnaire reached the goal set by the therapist. The differences in percentage between those returning and not returning the questionnaire on these two scales were significant for females ($p < 0.05$) but not for males. Females returning the questionnaire also reached or exceeded the therapists' goals on the *Problems* scale more frequently

Table 2–25
Percentage of Cases in which Therapists' Closing-Status Ratings
Reached or Exceeded Opening Goals

Scale	Clients Returning CSQ		Clients Not Returning CSQ	
	Males	Females	Males	Females
Family Interaction	56.8%	65.5%	54.8%	63.8%
Occupation	68.2	74.1	57.1	72.4
Getting Along with Others	63.6	77.6	64.3	72.4
Feelings and Mood	54.6	67.2	54.7	67.2
Use of Free Time	59.1	65.5[a]	45.3	44.8[a]
Problems	59.1	70.7[a]	61.9	51.7[a]
Attitude toward Self	61.1	69.8[a]	45.2	44.8[a]
Total score	47.7[a]	41.4	23.8[a]	27.6

[a]Percentages differ significantly, $p < 0.05$.

(70.7 percent) than did those not returning the questionnaire (51.7 percent). This difference was also significant. Comparing the percentage whose total closing adjustment score reached or exceeded therapists' summed goal ratings, it can be seen in the two sets of samples that both males and females returning the questionnaire were the higher. The difference is significant for males taken separately and for males and females combined.

In addition to giving some indication of the usefulness of the PES in assessing therapeutic outcome, these data lend support to claims that those returning consumer satisfaction questionnaires tend to be clients who benefited more from treatment than those who do not return the questionnaire.

Another analysis made possible by these data was the computation of correlations between the closing-status ratings made by the therapist and those made by the patient. These correlations were obtained for males and females separately and are shown in table 2–26. In table 2–26, the italicized values are correlations between corresponding scales. Nine of these 14 coefficents are above 0.30, indicating reasonably good convergence. The average correlation between corresponding scales is 0.32 for females and 0.37 for males. However, in some cases, higher correlations are found between different scales than between corresponding scales, particularly for the men. Thus, the therapists' ratings of *Occupational* adjustment, *Getting Along with Others, Feelings and Mood,* and *Attitude toward Self* are all more highly related to *Family Interaction* as rated by the male patient than is the therapist rating of *Family Interaction*. The latter rating corresponds more closely to what the men rate as *Getting Along with Others*. Ratings of *Feelings and Mood* by both the males and

Table 2–26
Correlations between Closing-Status Ratings of Therapist and Outpatients

		Patient Rating					
Scale	1	2	3	4	5	6	7
Females (N = 58)							
1 Family Interaction	26	22	23	19	09	23	19
2 Occupation	15	*41*	28	14	08	23	17
3 Getting Along with Others	−05	04	*40*	21	24	21	23
4 Feelings and Mood	07	10	19	*26*	18	33	25
5 Use of Free Time	−18	−05	06	03	*22*	07	04
6 Problems	10	12	21	25	38	*36*	22
7 Attitude toward Self	18	06	37	36	40	34	*31*
Males (N = 44)							
1 Family interaction	*18*	17	49	17	18	35	20
2 Occupation	46	*55*	49	23	24	46	47
3 Getting Along with Others	46	31	*32*	14	15	25	33
4 Feelings and Mood	45	37	29	*22*	31	33	34
5 Use of Free Time	35	22	32	23	*41*	38	37
6 Problems	22	05	34	24	21	*41*	30
7 Attitude toward Self	46	33	45	38	27	49	*47*

Note: Italicized values are correlations between corresponding scales. Decimal points are omitted.

females are more highly related to the therapists' ratings of *Attitude toward Self* than to their ratings of *Feelings and Mood*.

The rather poor discriminating power of the PES scales revealed in these closing ratings may be a function of the high correlations among scales as rated by both therapists and patients. These intercorrelations are displayed in table 2–27. The average intercorrelation among ratings of the therapists is 0.48 for females and 0.51 for males. Those for the patients are 0.44 and 0.46, respectively. These intercorrelations are considerably higher than were obtained among opening-status ratings. Such increases in intercorrelation from initial to final scores have been noted previously in the literature in connection with multiple-scored inventories and ratings (see Green, Gleser, Stone and Seifert 1975). It appears to be due to a tendency for both patients and therapists to perceive improvement globally, so that patients' ratings tend to dichotomize into those improved and those unimproved symptomatically and behaviorally.

Three-Month Reevaluation: A particularly interesting set of data was obtained on 42 adults for whom three-month goals were set and who were then reevaluated after three months in treatment by both therapist and patient. The sample consisted of 15 males and 27 females, ranging in age from 18 to 80 ($\overline{X}$ = 37.2, sd = 13.9). Twelve of the patients had neurotic problems, 18 had problems of adjustment, and 4 each were

Table 2–27
Intercorrelations among PES Scales for Closing-Status Ratings by Therapist and Patient on Male and Female Outpatients

Scale	Therapist						Patient					
	2	3	4	5	6	7	2	3	4	5	6	7
Females (N = 58)												
1 Family Interaction	54	38	42	37	42	27	45	37	53	23	49	32
2 Occupation		50	27	40	35	32		29	47	22	36	26
3 Getting Along with Others			64	67	54	59			57	54	55	41
4 Feelings and Mood				53	61	53				51	69	64
5 Use of Free Time					55	47					44	39
6 Problems						74						59
7 Attitude toward Self												
Males (N = 44)												
1 Family Interaction	44	31	31	23	51	32	66	57	46	35	55	17
2 Occupation		53	64	41	44	59		52	52	36	46	36
3 Getting Along with Others			59	60	48	60			56	60	56	30
4 Feelings and Mood				53	67	43				52	57	42
5 Use of Free Time					75	56					42	31
6 Problems						74						34
7 Attitude toward Self												

Note: Decimal points are omitted.

categorized as psychotic, personality disorder, or other. All but 11 were high-school graduates or better.

The mean status and goal ratings for patient and therapist, initially and at three months, are presented in table 2–28. A perusal of these means reveals that for these patients, the most-crucial problem areas are indicated by the last four scales. Their *Attitude toward Self* was primarily negative; they complained of almost continuous *Problems,* felt nervous, depressed, or angry for days at a time *(Feelings and Mood),* and made poor *Use of Free Time.* On three of these four scales, considerable improvement was made by the end of three months. For the other three scales, less improvement is noted, but judging by the goals, less change was expected.

Goals for the next six months appear to be changed only minimally from the initial ones. The therapist thought that problem areas could be further reduced; the patient hoped to improve further *Feelings and Mood* and *Attutide toward Self.* The correlations between the two sets of reevaluation goals ranged from 0.17 for *Occupation* to 0.45 for *Use of Free Time.*

While initial three-month goals of both therapist and patient are obviously somewhat optimistic compared to the status at reevaluation, nevertheless there is a fairly high relationship between the two sets of ratings in both cases. The therapist's goals correlated 0.31 to 0.53 with re-

Table 2–28
Means and Standard Deviations of Initial and Reevaluation Status Ratings and Goals for an Adult Sample (N = 42)

| | | Therapist | | | | Patient | | | |
| | | Initial | | Reevaluation | | Initial | | Reevaluation | |
Scale		Status	Goal	Status	Goal	Status	Goal	Status	Goal
Family Interaction	$\overline{X}$	3.74	4.45	3.88	4.45	3.79	4.50	4.02	4.64
	sd	.70	.74	.89	.59	.98	.74	1.00	.73
Occupation	$\overline{X}$	3.93	4.64	4.00	4.55	4.00	4.69	4.10	4.79
	sd	.89	.53	1.01	.50	.94	.72	1.21	.56
Getting Along with Others	$\overline{X}$	3.83	4.26	3.74	4.31	4.12	4.62	4.21	4.64
	sd	.99	.73	.94	.64	.83	.73	.78	.53
Feelings and Mood	$\overline{X}$	3.05	4.26	3.40	4.24	3.10	4.48	3.76	4.71
	sd	1.01	.66	1.01	.76	1.27	.94	1.19	.51
Use of Free Time	$\overline{X}$	2.98	4.12	3.02	4.12	2.10	4.55	3.17	4.43
	sd	1.24	.89	1.22	.80	1.39	.92	1.27	.94
Problems	$\overline{X}$	2.64	3.90	3.07	4.14	2.90	4.31	3.36	4.38
	sd	1.06	.73	1.05	.78	1.21	.95	1.14	.73
Attitude toward Self	$\overline{X}$	2.71	3.98	3.10	3.95	2.57	4.21	3.19	4.36
	sd	1.13	.87	1.01	.79	1.21	.90	1.17	.85

evaluation status, with a median of 0.38; those of the patient correlated 0.26 to 0.62 with reevaluation status, with a median of 0.39. The new goals of therapist and patient are correlated to about the same extent (median = 0.37).

The correlations between therapist and patient status ratings initially and at reevaluation are shown in table 2–29. For four of seven scales, the correlation between ratings of therapist and patient increased at reevaluation over that for the initial ratings. The median correlation at reevaluation is 0.59 and that initially is 0.57, so the two sets are fairly comparable. The median correlation between initial and reevaluation status is 0.46 for the therapists and 0.50 for the patients.

Ratings for the 12 neurotic patients were compared with those for the 18 cases diagnosed as adjustment reaction. Initially the neurotics were significantly more disturbed than the adjustment reactions on *Feelings and Mood* and *Attitude toward Self* ratings of both patient and therapist. They were less disturbed than were the adjustment reactions on *Family Interaction* and *Problems* according to the therapist, whereas the patients rated themselves as more disturbed. On all four scales, the neurotic patients saw themselves as more improved after three months than did the adjustment reactions. The therapists, on the other hand, recorded greater gains for the adjustment reactions in the areas of *Family Interaction* and *Problems*. Thus, the two groups of patients were much more similar at reassessment than they had been initially.

Conclusion

The average variance of therapists' status ratings on the PES scales, taking into account both differences among therapists and occasions of rating, is estimated to be 0.52. Further analyses indicate that 90 percent of the time a therapist's rating on these scales will be within 0.50 units from that obtainable were a large number of therapists to make ratings on the same individual on occasions spread out over a two-week interval. A difference of 0.4 between observed means of two groups of as few as 10 clients, each rated by different therapists, is reliable at the 90 percent level of confidence. Furthermore, a difference of one unit on a scale, rated by the same therapist or client on two occasions, represents a real change at the 90 percent level of confidence.

Initial-status ratings on the seven scales are positively intercorrelated to a low or moderate degree in both nonpatient and patient samples. Thus, while a common factor of overall adjustment appears indicated, the individual scales also yield considerable independent information. Goal ratings are considerably more highly intercorrelated than are status ratings.

Table 2–29
Correlations between Initial Status and Reevaluation Ratings of Therapists and Patients (N = 42)

	Therapist Reevaluation	Patient Evaluation	Patient Reevaluation
Family Interaction			
Therapist			
Evaluation	0.46	0.17	0.18
Reevaluation		.45	.44
Patient evaluation			.36
Occupation			
Therapist			
Evaluation	.56	.58	.37
Reevaluation		.41	.80
Patient evaluation			.47
Getting Along with Others			
Therapist			
Evaluation	.22	.56	.08
Reevaluation		.23	.48
Patient evaluation			.56
Feelings and Mood			
Therapist			
Evaluation	.31	.49	.17
Reevaluation		.24	.59
Patient evaluation			.49
Use of Free Time			
Therapist			
Evaluation	.50	.62	.30
Reevaluation		.53	.61
Patient evaluation			.74
Problems			
Therapist			
Evaluation	.44	.57	.45
Reevaluation		.35	.51
Patient evaluation			.59
Attitude toward Self			
Therapist			
Evaluation	.60	.51	.41
Reevaluation		.47	.73
Patient evaluation			.50

Initial-status ratings of clients and their therapists are highly and significantly correlated, with an average correlation of 0.48 between ratings on the same scale. Correlations between ratings of different scales are all lower than those obtained on corresponding scales, indicating that valid discriminations are being made with regard to the underlying dimensions.

Self-ratings of initial status on the PES significantly differentiate normal groups of males and females from physically handicapped individuals; both sets of ratings differ significantly from self-ratings of clients seen in a community mental-health center.

PES initial-status and goal ratings are not determined to any extent by demographic variables. Relatively few significant correlations were obtained between ratings and such variables as age, sex, marital status, and income. Occupational status as rated by both therapist and client was higher for males who were older and had a higher income. For females, higher income was correlated with better family interaction. Differences occurring between initial-status ratings of male and female clients in some samples appeared to be due to sampling fluctuations.

Diagnostic groupings can be differentiated by PES ratings. Neurotics scored higher, on the average, than psychotics on all scales except *Feelings and Mood*. Clients having adjustment reactions scored higher on several scales than did those classified as neurotics or personality disorder. Also clients classified as having personality disorders tended to rate themselves higher on a number of scales than did their therapists. Differences among the groups on goal setting were also noted.

The PES scales are sensitive to changes in status. Ratings at termination or reevaluation were investigated in three studies. In all three, average ratings increased relative to initial scores but did not reach initial goals, according to both therapist and client. Goals on separate scales were reached, however, for well over half the clients. Clients who returned a consumer satisfaction questionnaire achieved somewhat greater improvement, according to their therapists' ratings, but they also tended to be rated somewhat higher initially. On reevaluation, clients tended to see themselves as better adjusted personally and socially than did their therapists.

3

Application of Progress Evaluation Scales to Children and Adolescents

Generalizability Studies

Observer-Rater Reliability

The extent to which therapists agree in their ratings of status and goals for children and adolescent outpatients was examined in an early study. A staff member sat in on the therapists's initial diagnostic interview and independently rated the client as to present status and three-month goals. Samples of 20 children aged 6 through 12 and 20 adolescents aged 13 through 18 were analyzed separately. Data for only the first six scales are available since the seventh scale, *Attitude toward Self,* had not yet been developed.

The mean profiles for children and adolescents as rated by each of the staff members are reported in table 3–1 and shown in figures 3–1 and 3–2. These profiles for current status and for goals are in fairly close agreement, with one or two exceptions. The only significant difference is in the scale *Use of Free Time,* with children, where the difference is 0.55.

The data were analyzed for each scale separately to obtain estimates of the amount of variance attributable to differences among clients ($\hat{\sigma}_p^2$) and that due to average differences between ratings of therapists on any one person ($\hat{\sigma}_e^2$). The ratio of ($\hat{\sigma}_p^2$) to the expected observed-score variance ($\hat{\sigma}_x^2$) yields an estimate of reliability (r_{xx}). These values are shown in table 3–1. This method of computing reliability takes into account the fact that in ordinary use of the scale, clients will be rated by different therapists. Therefore therapists' mean score differences will contribute to error variance. Such estimates, however, tend to be lower than those obtained by correlating the two sets of scores, since the latter method ignores differences among therapists' means.

As indicated in table 3–1, reliability estimates for current status range from 0.14 for *Use of Free Time* to a high of 0.82 for *Getting Along with Others,* both occurring in the children's sample. The median reliabilities were 0.47 for children and 0.44 for adolescents. The corresponding median reliabilities for goals were 0.40 and 0.50. The reliabilities for goals

Table 3–1
Comparison of Two Therapists' Ratings on Children and Adolescent Psychiatric Samples of Twenty Patients Each

Scale	Children						Adolescents					
	M_{t_1}	M_{t_2}	$\hat{\sigma}_x^2$	$\hat{\sigma}_p^2$	$\hat{\sigma}_e^2$	r_{xx}	M_{t_1}	M_{t_2}	$\hat{\sigma}_x^2$	$\hat{\sigma}_p^2$	$\hat{\sigma}_e^2$	r_{xx}
Family Interaction												
Present	3.95	3.90	0.73	0.41	0.32	0.56	3.90	3.75	0.35	0.13	0.22	0.38
Goal	4.40	4.40	.45	.10	.35	.23	4.30	4.25	.36	.04	.32	.10
Occupation												
Present	3.95	4.10	.92	.64	.28	.69	3.20	3.50	.97	.67	.30	.69
Goal	4.40	4.60	.36	.21	.15	.60	3.95	4.10	.70	.48	.22	.69
Getting Along with Others												
Present	3.85	3.70	.97	.79	.18	.82	3.75	4.00	1.16	.68	.48	.58
Goal	4.45	4.30	.43	.15	.28	.35	4.10	4.45	.73	.41	.32	.56
Feelings and Mood												
Present	3.65	3.80	.67	.25	.42	.37	2.95	3.10	1.12	.54	.58	.48
Goal	4.55	4.35	.62	.27	.35	.44	4.05	3.85	.78	.38	.40	.48
Use of Free Time												
Present	3.55	4.10	.61	.09	.52	.14	3.50	3.75	1.23	.45	.78	.37
Goal	4.45	4.40	.51	.18	.22	.36	4.10	4.25	.56	.08	.48	.15
Problems												
Present	3.60	3.05	.50	.18	.32	.36	3.05	3.00	.70	.28	.42	.39
Goal	4.45	4.35	.56	.31	.25	.55	4.00	3.75	.58	.30	.28	.52

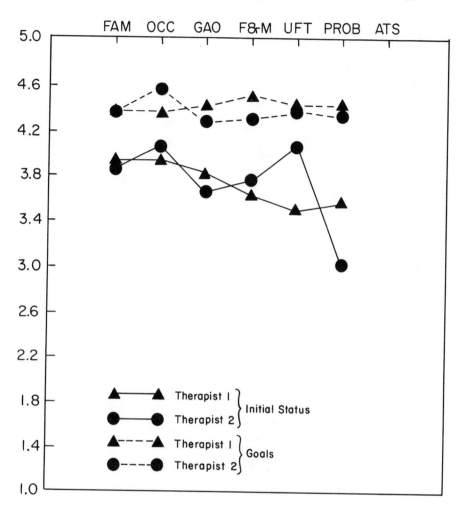

Figure 3–1. Comparison of Two Therapists' Ratings for Initial Status
and Goals for Sample of Twenty Children Outpatients

are comparable to those obtained with adults, but those for current status
are somewhat lower.

A more-recent estimate of the reliability of ratings over observers,
using the current seven scales, was obtained on a sample of severely
disturbed children in a day-treatment setting (day hospital). These children
were evaluated independently by the staff (5 to 7 people) on the PES
scales after one to six months in the program. Fourteen children, aged
6 to 16, were thus evaluated. Their mean profile, computed on averaged

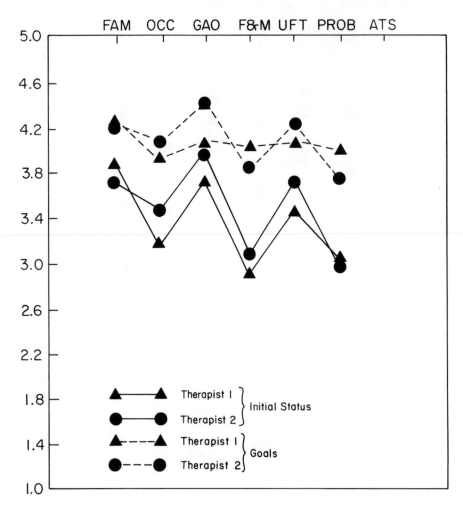

Figure 3–2. Comparison of Two Therapists' Ratings for Initial Status
and Goals for Sample of Twenty Adolescent Outpatients

ratings for each child, and the estimated variance components attributable to clients and to error are shown in table 3–2 for ratings of present status and goals. A comparison with the children's data in table 3–1 indicates that these children are much more poorly adjusted on all dimensions than are the outpatients seen in the Shiawassee County Mental Health Center.

The estimated variances among raters ($\hat{\sigma}_e^2$) are quite comparable for the two samples for ratings of current status, ranging from 0.18 to 0.52 in the outpatient sample and 0.18 to 0.50 for the day hospital. The median estimate of error variance is 0.32 for the outpatients versus 0.41 for the

Table 3–2
Estimates of True Score and Error Variances for PES Scales Used with a Sample of Disturbed Children in a Day-Treatment Center (N = 14)

Scale	Present Rating				Goals			
	$M_{\bar{x}}$	$\hat{\sigma}_p^2$	$\hat{\sigma}_e^2$	$\hat{r}_{xx}$	$M_{\bar{x}}$	$\hat{\sigma}_p^2$	$\hat{\sigma}_e^2$	$\hat{r}_{xx}$
Family Interaction	2.54	0.53	0.18	0.74	3.12	0.29	0.44	0.40
Occupation	2.25	.45	.46	.50	2.81	.53	.52	.50
Getting Along with Others	2.33	.25	.37	.41	3.00	.32	.38	.45
Feelings and Mood	2.13	.17	.50	.26	2.84	.19	.75	.20
Use of Free Time	2.14	.36	.49	.42	2.86	.34	.59	.37
Problems	1.83	.33	.41	.44	2.40	.30	.41	.42
Attitudes toward Self	1.78	.15	.23	.40	2.55	.18	.42	.30

day hospital. Estimated variance among raters for goal ratings is slightly higher in the day hospital than in the outpatient sample, yielding a median of 0.44 as compared to 0.30. The scale *Use of Free Time* again has a relatively high error variance, second only to *Feelings and Mood* for both current status and goals.

The estimated reliability of ratings by any one observer is indicated in the column headed r_{xx}. The median coefficients for the day-hospital sample are 0.42 and 0.40 for present status and goals, respectively. These correspond closely to the coefficients obtained for the outpatient sample. That these coefficients are low is primarily attributable to the restricted ranges involved in each sample. That they are restricted is evident by the sizable differences in average scale scores for the outpatients as compared to the day-hospital sample. Estimates of error variance present the clearest picture. Combining all available data, the average error variance for ratings of present status is approximately 0.36, yielding a standard error of measurement of 0.6. Thus, one can say that 90 percent of the time, ratings on some one scale would be 1 point or less from the "true" score (that is, the score that would be obtained if a large number of ratings were made on the same client at the same point in time).

Although the variances among ratings of children were not much larger than those for adults averaged over all scales, there did appear to be unduly large rater variance on some scales. This difficulty in obtaining reliable ratings among therapists for children after a one-hour diagnostic interview led to a reconsideration of our intake procedures for this population. The source of the difficulty appears to lie in the fact that children's behavior is often difficult to interpret since few of their problems are given verbal expression and, more importantly, parental reports are frequently inconsistent. To improve the quality of data gathering for this population, ratings of children on the PES are now made after two or three intake sessions. In these sessions, the interviewer gets better acquainted with each parent, resolves inconsistent reports, and evaluates more closely the child's behavior and personality.

Stability over Occasions

A sample of 17 children was analyzed for whom the mother and father filled out ratings of present status at the time the child was screened for possible service and approximately two weeks later at the completion of the diagnostic interview. Similar data were also obtained on two occasions for 18 adolescents, with ratings by the adolescent and his or her mother. Estimated variance components were obtained for client, occasions, and the interaction of client and occasion for a given rater. These are shown in table 3–3.

Table 3–3
Generalizability of PES Present Status over Occasions for Children and Adolescents

	Children[a] (N = 17)				Adolescents[b] (N = 18)			
Scale	$\hat{\sigma}_p^2$	$\hat{\sigma}_o^2$	$\hat{\sigma}_{po,e}^2$	r_{xx}	$\hat{\sigma}_p^2$	$\hat{\sigma}_o^2$	$\hat{\sigma}_{po,e}^2$	r_{xx}
Family Interaction	0.85	0.01	0.34	0.72	0.47	0.00	0.27	0.64
Occupation	.66	.00	.37	.64	.93	.00	.83	.53
Getting Along with Others	1.08	.00	.37	.75	1.09	.02	.69	.61
Feelings and Mood	1.00	.00	.43	.70	1.30	.00	.79	.62
Use of Free Time	.58	.00	.96	.38	.93	.07	.86	.50
Problems	.54	.00	.29	.65	.73	.04	.38	.63
Attitude to Self	.33	.00	.67	.33	.43	.00	.76	.36

[a]Ratings by mother or by father.
[b]Ratings by client or by mother.

For the children there was no systematic change from screening to diagnostic interview on any of the scales as indicated by the zero values for ($\hat{\sigma}_o^2$). However, adolescents on the average had increased ratings in *Getting Along with Others, Use of Free Time,* and *Problems* at the time of the diagnostic interview as compared to their initial ratings ($\hat{\sigma}_o^2 > o$). Ratings on individuals differed considerably from one occasion to another; the estimated variance components for clients × occasions ($\hat{\sigma}_{po,e}^2$) ranging from 0.29 to 0.96 for children and 0.27 to 0.86 for adolescents. For both groups the least-stable ratings were for *Use of Free Time* and the most stable for *Problems* and *Family Interaction.* The estimated reliability coefficients ranged from 0.33 to 0.75, with a median of 0.65 for children and 0.61 for adolescents.

Correlations between Current Status and Three-Month Goals

Another interesting relationship among ratings is that between the goals set by one therapist and the initial status ratings of another therapist. These are correlations between independent ratings whereas the correlations usually obtained between goals and status ratings of a single therapist are inflated by correlated error. These latter correlations have been designated as linked (Cronbach et al. 1972).

The linked and independent correlations between present status and goal ratings for pairs of therapist raters in 20 children and 20 adolescents are displayed in table 3–4. As expected, the linked correlations are higher than the independent correlations for all scales, indicating the extent to which error of measurement for current functioning and goals are interdependent. The unlinked correlations range from 0.20 for *Use of Free*

Table 3–4

Correlations between Current Status and Three-Month Goals as Rated by Two Therapists on Children and Adolescent Samples

Scale	Children (N = 20)		Adolescent (N = 20)	
	Linked (Same Therapist)	Independent	Linked (Same Therapist)	Independent
Family Interaction	0.72	0.42	0.43	0.22
Occupation	.70	.55	.83	.64
Getting Along with Others	.72	.66	.87	.57
Feelings and Mood	.73	.52	.70	.33
Use of Free Time	.52	.32	.80	.20
Problems	.64	.29	.78	.38

Time in adolescents to 0.66 for *Getting Along with Others* in children, with a median of 0.40.

Construct Validity Studies

Comparisons of Central Tendencies and Deviations from the Means for Normative and Patient Populations

Means and Standard Deviations on Nonpatient Samples: Samples of ratings of current functioning on the PES have been obtained from several nonpatient groups of boys and girls. The largest of these groups, consisting of 53 male and 157 female white adolescents, came from high-school classes in Shiawassee County, Michigan. The adolescents rated themselves on the PES. Scores for 18 boys and 18 girls were obtained by asking parents attending a PTA meeting to rate their children on these scales. No identifying information was requested except age, sex, and educational level. Means and standard deviations of status scores on the seven scales are displayed in table 3–5.

Like the adults, the adolescents rate themselves higher on the first four scales than on the last three. The girls rate themselves higher on *Family Interaction, Getting Along with Others,* and *Problems* than do the boys. Interestingly the adolescents rate themselves lower on the PES than do the adults. The adolescent males are significantly lower than adult males on all scales except *Feelings and Mood;* the female adolescents are significantly lower for all but *Getting Along with Others, Use of Free Time,* and *Problems.* The children have better scores on *Use of Free Time* and *Problems* than do the adolescents.

Table 3–5
Means and Standard Deviations of PES Scores for Samples of
Normally Functioning Male and Female Adolescents and Children

Scale	Adolescent[a]		Children[b]	
	Male (N = 53)	Female (N = 157)	Male (N = 18)	Female (N = 18)
Age				
$\overline{X}$	14.1	15.3	9.4	8.6
sd	2.0	2.0	1.8	1.9
Family Interaction				
$\overline{X}$	4.13	4.40	4.06	4.00
sd	.94	.86	.87	.84
Occupation				
$\overline{X}$	4.58	4.50	4.67	4.78
sd	.72	.81	.59	.43
Getting Along with Others				
$\overline{X}$	4.19	4.65	4.33	4.50
sd	1.27	.69	.84	.62
Feelings and Mood				
$\overline{X}$	4.51	4.39	4.44	4.67
sd	.72	.88	1.04	.49
Use of Free Time				
$\overline{X}$	3.83	3.87	4.17	4.50
sd	.91	1.09	.99	.79
Problems				
$\overline{X}$	3.87	4.19	4.72	4.56
sd	1.07	.99	.46	.62
Attitude toward Self				
$\overline{X}$	3.85	3.71	4.17	4.11
sd	1.01	1.15	.92	.83

[a]Self-ratings.
[b]Ratings by mother.

Comparison of Normal and Patient Groups: An important reason for obtaining data on normative samples is to compare them with data obtained on various patient populations that can be expected to differ from nonpatients on the variables measured by the PES. Samples of 20 girls and 39 boys seen in the outpatient service of the Shiawassee Mental Health Center in 1977 were drawn sequentially in order of admittance. All of these children had been rated on the PES for current status by their mothers. Data on samples of 16 girls and 33 boys were obtained from partial-hospitalization programs operated in three different counties in Michigan. These three programs were similar to each other. The children in each program were rated by their therapists who knew them for from six months to two years. Finally, 18 girls and 61 boys, consisting of Shiawassee County children enrolled in emotionally impaired classes, were each rated by their teacher. The means for each of these groups are displayed in table 3–6.

Table 3–6
Means and Standard Deviations of PES Scores by Sex for Samples of Children from Three Populations

Scale	Male			Female		
	Outpatients (N = 39)	Emotionally Impaired (N = 61)	Partial Hospitalization (N = 33)	Outpatients (N = 20)	Emotionally Impaired (N = 18)	Partial Hospitalization (N = 16)
Family Interaction						
$\overline{X}$	3.28	3.67	2.76	3.20	3.77	3.00
sd	.86	.87	1.12	.89	.65	.73
Occupation						
$\overline{X}$	4.08	3.93	2.30	4.00	3.94	1.94
sd	1.09	.83	1.19	1.08	.80	1.06
Getting Along with Others						
$\overline{X}$	3.18	3.15	2.12	2.80	3.44	2.00
sd	1.05	1.05	.93	.62	.92	.73
Feelings and Mood						
$\overline{X}$	3.46	3.48	2.36	3.00	3.27	1.75
sd	1.17	1.12	.96	1.34	1.27	.74
Use of Free Time						
$\overline{X}$	3.28	3.11	2.36	2.90	3.22	2.31
sd	1.26	.95	.96	1.33	1.06	1.08
Problems						
$\overline{X}$	3.44	3.38	1.94	3.15	3.38	1.63
sd	.99	1.16	.83	1.04	1.29	.72
Attitude toward Self						
$\overline{X}$	2.66	2.87	1.67	2.90	2.83	1.50
sd	.85	1.09	.60	1.02	1.10	.63

Note: Outpatient groups were rated by their mothers; children in emotionally impaired classes were rated by their teachers; children in partial hospitalization were rated by their therapists who knew the children for six months to two years.

Figures 3–3 and 3–4 compare the profiles of the patient samples to those for the normal children. It is quite obvious that the PES scales sharply differentiate both male and female samples. The partial-hospitalization groups differ significantly from the outpatient group and those attending classes for the emotionally impaired. These last two groups have similar profiles, which differ markedly and significantly from those of the normative children.

A similar comparison among normative and patient samples was

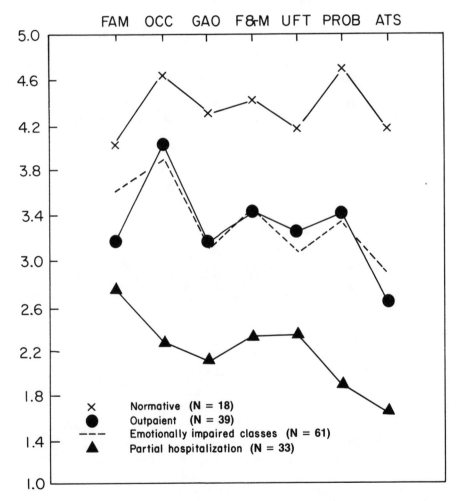

Figure 3–3. Comparison of Normative Boys to Boys Seen in Outpatient Services, Emotionally Impaired Classes, and Partial Hospitalization

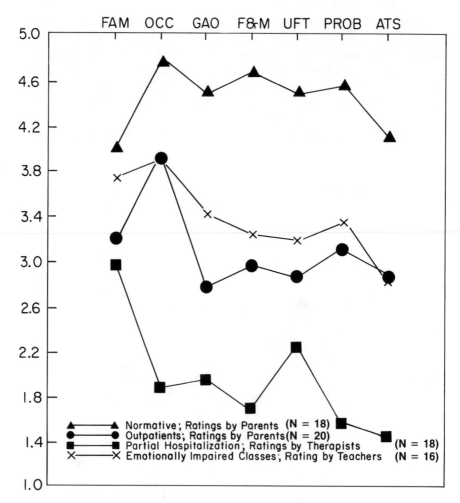

Figure 3–4. Comparison of Normative Girls to Girls Seen in Outpatient Services, Emotionally Impaired Classes, and Partial Hospitalization

obtained for adolescents. Samples of 50 females and 50 males were selected from outpatients seen at the Shiawassee County Mental Health Center in 1977, all of whom had been rated on initial status on the PES scales by their therapists. Additionally, 10 male adolescents from classes for emotionally impaired were rated by their teachers, and 30 adolescent males and 8 adolescent females in partial-hospitalization programs were rated by their therapists. The means and standard deviations of scores for these samples are shown in table 3–7. These profiles are compared in

Table 3–7
Means and Standard Deviations of PES Scores by Sex for Samples of Adolescents from Three Populations

Scale	Male			Female	
	Outpatients (N = 50)	Emotionally Impaired (N = 10)	Partial Hospitalization (N = 30)	Outpatients (N = 50)	Partial Hospitalization (N = 8)
Family Interaction					
$\overline{X}$	3.46	3.40	2.93	3.56	2.87
sd	.68	.70	.83	.58	.84
Occupation					
$\overline{X}$	3.14	3.50	2.63	3.62	2.25
sd	1.24	.85	1.22	1.32	1.04
Getting Along with Others					
$\overline{X}$	3.68	3.00	2.63	3.88	2.00
sd	1.11	1.05	.67	.92	.76
Feelings and Mood					
$\overline{X}$	3.36	3.60	2.17	3.08	1.86
sd	1.08	1.07	.83	.88	.99
Use of Free Time					
$\overline{X}$	3.40	3.40	2.47	3.22	2.13
sd	1.03	1.07	.94	1.15	.83
Problems					
$\overline{X}$	2.90	3.90	1.87	2.76	1.75
sd	.84	.99	.68	.87	.87
Attitude toward Self					
$\overline{X}$	2.90	2.70	1.77	2.78	1.50
sd	1.02	.82	.63	1.00	.76

Note: Emotionally impaired were rated by their teachers; partial hospitalization and outpatient clients were rated by their primary therapist.

figures 3–5 and 3–6 to those of a small normative sample of adolescents (18 males and 14 females) rated by their mothers. For these samples, as for the children, the profiles are sharply differentiated in the expected direction.

Relationship of PES Scales to Demographic Variables
and Measures of Adjustment and Personality

Although the majority of the data collected on the PES scales has come from Shiawassee County, Michigan, we have also been able to obtain

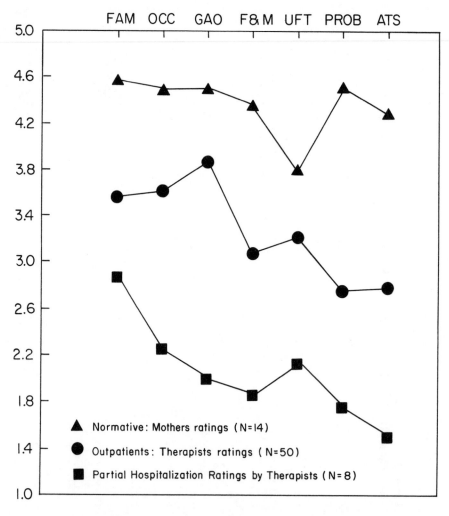

Figure 3–5. Comparison of Normative Female Adolescents to Outpatients and Adolescents in Partial Hospitalization

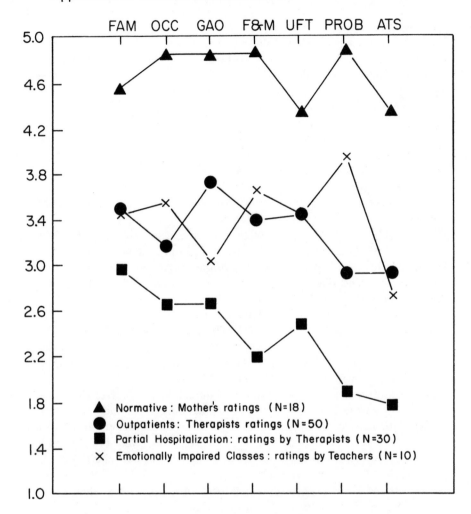

Figure 3–6. Comparison of Normative Male Adolescents to Outpatients, Adolescents in Partial Hospitalization, and Those Enrolled in Emotionally Impaired Classes

data on normative adolescents from a large urban center, Cincinnati, Ohio. PES scores on 112 adolescents were obtained in the summer of 1975 as part of a larger study to obtain normative data on a number of instruments for use with adolescents. In addition to the PES, the Adolescent Life Assessment Checklist (ALAC), the Defense Mechanisms Inventory (DMI), and Rotter's I-E Scale were administered to volunteers stratified with respect to sex, race, and age.

The 56 boys and 56 girls were solicited through the Commission for Youth from the Rent-a-Kid and similar programs. The youngest group,

11 and 12 years of age, was obtained from summer playgrounds. The children were each paid six dollars to participate.

The research design was a three-factor, crossed design consisting of an equal number of blacks, whites, males, and females from four age levels: 11–12, 13–14, 15–16, and 17–18. Thus, there were sixteen cells in all, with seven children per cell. Table 3–8 summarizes the means by sex and race and separately by age.

Highly significant differences (p <0.001) were found between black and white adolescents in their evaluation of *Occupation* and *Use of Free Time*. On both these scales the black adolescents rated themselves lower than did the white. They also rated themselves as somewhat poorer at *Getting Along with Others* (p = 0.06). There were no significant differences for sex, but for two scales the race-sex interactions were significant. The black females saw themselves as having more *Problems* than did the white females or the males of both races (P = 0.01). The black females also had the poorest *Attitude toward Self*, followed by the white males. The black males were most positive about themselves of the four groups (p = 0.04).

Age differences were found for *Family Interaction* (p = 0.01) and for *Feelings and Mood* (p = 0.05). The ratings for *Family Interaction* increased steadily with age. The trend for *Feelings and Mood* was more irregular, the peak occurring for the 13 to 14 year olds, whereas the lowest ratings were made by the 11 to 12 year olds.

In addition to age, race, and sex of the adolescents, data were available on birth order, number of siblings, and educational and occupational level of the head of the household. Pearson-product-moment correlations revealed no relation between birth order or number of siblings and the self-evaluations. The educational level of the head of household did relate negatively, however, with *Occupation* (r = −0.23) and *Problems* (r = −0.26). Evidently the children from more highly educated families tended to see themselves as having more difficulty in school (since this is their primary occupation) and as being troubled with more problems.

The ALAC, a self-report inventory (Gleser et al. 1977), provides scores on six subscales dealing with *Affective Distress, Unproductivity, Sociopathy, Peer Alienation, Somatic Complaints*, and *Tolerance of Intimacy*. All but the last scale are keyed so that a higher score indicates more pathology. Thus, correlations between the PES and the first five scales were expected to be negative, whereas those for *Tolerance of Intimacy* were expected to be positive.

The correlations obtained between the PES and the ALAC for the entire sample are shown in table 3–9. A number of highly significant correlations emerged. *Family Interaction* correlated 0.26 with *Tolerance of Intimacy*. Poor *Occupation* (school adjustment) related significantly

Table 3-8
Mean Self-Evaluations of Adolescents Summarized by Sex and Race and by Age (N = 28)

	Family Interaction		Occupation		Getting Along		Feelings and Mood		Use of Free Time		Problems		Attitude to Self	
	Black	White	Black	White	Black	White	Black	White	Black	White	Black	White	Black	White
By sex and race														
Females	3.48[a]	3.89	3.89[a]	4.68	4.15[a]	4.57	4.19[a]	4.36	3.52[a]	4.36	3.33[a]	4.36	3.33[a]	3.82
Males	3.71	3.85[a]	4.11	4.70	4.11	4.28	4.00	4.21	3.57	4.36	4.25	4.11	4.14	3.75
Total	3.60	3.87	4.00	4.59	4.13	4.42	4.10	4.28	3.54	4.36	3.84	4.24	3.74	3.78
By age														
11–12	3.11[a]		4.15[a]		4.21[a]		3.67[a]		3.46[a]		3.71[a]		3.58[a]	
13–14	3.59		4.48		4.16		4.63		4.26		4.39		3.93	
15–16	3.89[a]		4.36		4.30		4.18		4.10		4.14		3.75	
17–18	4.32		4.36		4.44		4.18		4.03		3.82		3.82	
Total	3.74		4.34		4.28		4.19		3.97		4.02		3.77	
sd within groups	1.34		.93		.97		1.10		1.24		1.26		1.08	
sd total	1.34		.98		.95		1.12		1.34		1.32		1.08	

[a]N = 27.

Table 3–9
Correlations between PES Scales and Adolescent Life Assessment Checklist (N = 105)

PES Scale	ALAC Scales[a]					
	Affective Distress	*Unproductivity*	*Sociopathy*	*Peer Alienation*	*Somatic Complaints*	*Tolerance of Intimacy*
Family Interaction	−0.13	−0.05	−0.13	−0.14	−0.03	0.26**
Occupation	−.14	−.24*	−.28**	−.32***	−.51***	.02
Getting Along with Others	−.12	−.07	−.20*	−.26**	−.01	.19
Feelings and Mood	−.42***	−.37***	−.43***	−.31**	−.22*	−.03
Use of Free Time	.01	−.07	−.14	−.31**	−.07	.30**
Problems	−.46***	−.39***	−.34***	−.27**	−.30**	−.04
Attitude toward Self	−.14	−.25*	−.25*	−.23*	−.14	.12

[a]For the first five scales a higher score indicates more pathology, whereas for the last scale a lower score is more pathological.

*$p \leq 0.05$.
**$p \leq 0.01$.
***$p \leq 0.001$.

with *Unproductivity* (−0.24), *Sociopathy* (−0.28), *Peer Alienation* (−0.32), and *Somatic Complaints* (−0.51). Difficulty in *Getting Along with Others* was associated with *Sociopathy* (−0.20), *Peer Alienation* (−0.26), and poor *Tolerance of Intimacy* (0.19). Poor *Use of Free Time* was also associated with *Peer Alienation* (−0.31) and poor *Tolerance of Intimacy* (0.30). Both *Feelings and Mood* and *Problems* correlated significantly with five of the six scales, the highest correlations obtaining for *Affective Distress, Unproductivity,* and *Sociopathy.* The convergence of these two methods of assessing adjustment indicates a high degree of concurrent validity for both instruments.

Additional data of interest are the correlations between the PES ratings and scores on the Defense Mechanisms Inventory (Gleser and Ihilevich 1969) and Rotter's I-E Scale (Rotter 1966). These are shown in table 3–10. The only scale that correlated significantly ($p<0.05$) with the I-E Scale was *Occupation.* The "internal reinforcers" saw themselves as functioning better in school than did those who were more "external." However, race was correlated with both the I-E scores and the occupational ratings. When this factor was controlled statistically, the partial correlation between I-E and *Occupation* (school) rating was −0.14, which is not significant. Since blacks have previously been shown to be more externally controlled than whites, this seems to be the most reasonable explanation of the significant zero-order correlation between I-E and *Occupational* rating. Other correlations of interest in table 3–10, from the construct validity standpoint, are the negative correlations between *Turning against Self* and *Family Interaction* (−0.22) and *Attitude toward Self* (−0.33), and the positive correlations between *Principalization* and *Family Interaction* (0.31) and *Getting Along with Others* (0.20). Youngsters who are more inclined to blame themselves tend to have low self-esteem and to be a burden on their families; people who use more intellectual defenses get along better both with their families and with peers, as might be expected.

Intercorrelations among PES Scale Self-Ratings

Intercorrelations were obtained among the self-ratings of three normative samples: the 157 girls and 53 boys from high schools in Shiawassee County, Michigan, and the normative sample of 105 boys and girls from Cincinnati on whom data were complete. These correlations are exhibited in table 3–11. The intercorrelations tend to be low, averaging 0.30 for girls, 0.16 for boys, and 0.22 for the mixed sample. The higher correlations for girls are similar to that seen for adult samples. Judging from these correlations, *Problems* for boys tend to be related more to school

Table 3–10
Correlations between PES Self-Evaluations and Defense Mechanisms Inventory and Rotter's Internal–External Control Scores for Normative Sample of Adolescents (N = 105)

Scale	Defense Mechanisms					Rotter's Internal/External Control
	Turning against Others	Projection	Principalization	Turning against Self	Reversal	
1 Family Interaction	−0.12	−0.02	0.31**	−0.22*	0.08	−0.09
2 Occupation	−.20*	−.10	.13	.05	.16	−.22*
3 Getting Along with Others	−.08	−.10	.20*	.02	.00	−.16
4 Feelings and Mood	−.06	−.10	.13	−.01	.05	−.07
5 Use of Free Time	−.08	−.06	.17	−.06	.07	−.03
6 Problems	−.03	.00	.13	−.08	.03	−.10
7 Attitude toward Self	.13	.07	.06	−.33**	.01	−.13

*$p \leq 0.05$.
**$p \leq 0.01$.

Table 3–11
Intercorrelations among Progress Evaluation Self-Ratings of
Normative Adolescent Samples

Scale	Girls (N = 157)						Boys (N = 53)					
	2	3	4	5	6	7	2	3	4	5	6	7
1 Family Interaction	31	37	23	25	33	31	05	−12	10	09	15	35
2 Occupation		17	22	21	35	33		40	12	21	40	11
3 Getting Along			35	29	33	33			23	04	40	16
4 Feelings and Mood				22	41	32				−30	26	29
5 Use of Free Time					23	42					−08	17
6 Problems						24						29
7 Attitude toward Self												

Scale	Black and White Boys and Girls (N = 105)					
	2	3	4	5	6	7
1 Family Interaction	04	14	25	20	26	26
2 Occupation		05	16	24	36	03
3 Getting Along			17	15	09	23
4 Feelings and Moods				32	40	37
5 Use of Free Time					31	30
6 Problems						25
7 Attitude toward Self						

Note: Decimal points are omitted.

adjustment *(Occupation)* and *Getting Along with Others*, whereas for girls this scale relates additionally with *Family Interaction* and *Feelings and Mood*.

Intercorrelations among self-ratings for the adolescent boys and girls seen in the outpatient service of the Shiawassee Mental Health Center are shown in table 3–12. These correlations are also low, averaging 0.36 for girls and 0.22 for boys. The higher intercorrelations for females are

Table 3–12
Intercorrelations among Initial-Status Self-Ratings of Adolescent
Outpatients

Scale	Males (N = 42)						Females (N = 41)					
	2	3	4	5	6	7	2	3	4	5	6	7
1 Family Interaction	23	−08	08	24	27	08	41	14	10	28	21	35
2 Occupation		09	20	26	22	05		35	48	41	29	42
3 Getting Along with Others			−04	11	14	45			47	54	18	38
4 Feelings and Mood				42	35	28				51	39	54
5 Use of Free Time					46	49					12	56
6 Problems						36						63
7 Attitude to Self												

Note: Decimal points are omitted.

again evident. The generally positive intercorrelations indicate that the scores on the separate scales could be summed to yield a scale of overall adjustment that might be useful in some outcome studies.

Studies of Therapy Outcome

Adolescents: In our first study of therapy outcome with adolescents, carried out before the seventh scale was devised, there were only 14 adolescents on whom termination ratings were available. These young-sters had all rated themselves on the PES at the beginning, whereas the therapist had rated them initially and at the time the case was closed. Eight of the sample were boys and 6 were girls. Half had been seen for only one or two sessions, with a range of from one to twenty-nine sessions. The average age of the group was 16.4 years, with a standard deviation of 2.6.

Data are summarized in table 3–13. The initial mean PES scores of therapist and patient are quite similar, with the largest difference, 0.29, occurring for *Occupation*. This was also the lowest score in the profile, probably indicating these youngsters were all having school problems. That these problems were not resolved seems indicated by their continued low score in this area at closing. However, they had improved a half-point or more, on the average, in *Feelings and Mood, Use of Free Time,* and in resolving the *Problems* for which they sought help. Their inter-action with the family apparently had also improved somewhat.

A larger sample of adolescents, consisting of 50 boys and 50 girls,

Table 3–13
Means and Standard Deviations of Initial and Closing PES Ratings on an Adolescent Sample (N = 14)

Scale		Opening		Closing
		Patient	Therapist	Therapist
Family Interaction	$\overline{X}$	3.50	3.28	3.71
	sd	.94	.82	.73
Occupation	$\overline{X}$	2.57	2.86	2.93
	sd	1.28	1.29	1.64
Getting Along with Others	$\overline{X}$	3.57	3.57	4.00
	sd	1.22	1.16	.96
Feelings and Mood	$\overline{X}$	3.36	3.43	4.07
	sd	1.50	.85	.83
Use of Free Time	$\overline{X}$	3.43	3.21	3.78
	sd	1.34	1.42	.97
Problems	$\overline{X}$	2.86	3.07	3.64
	sd	1.17	1.07	.74

was available by 1977. Average age for these groups was 15.5 for the boys and 15.7 for the girls. Means and standard deviations for initial PES status and goals as rated by therapists, patients, and parents are shown in table 3.14 for males and table 3–15 for females. Comparisons among both initial status and goal ratings are also illustrated in figures 3–7 and 3–8 for those youngsters on whom all three ratings were available (males, N = 26; females, N = 20). The profiles for the three sets of ratings are highly similar. However, it is interesting that the adolescents' current-

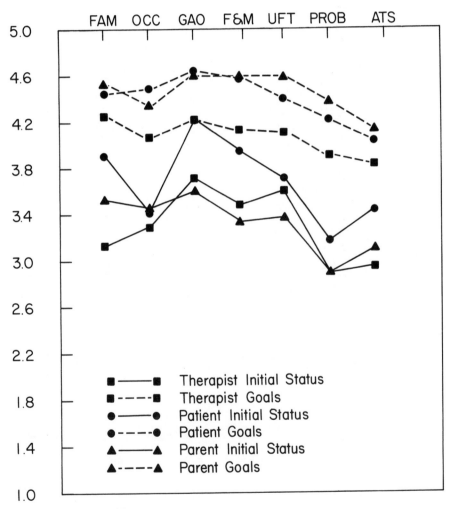

Figure 3–7. Comparison of Initial Ratings by Therapist, Patient, and Parent on Twenty-six Male Adolescents

Table 3–14
Means and Standard Deviations for PES Opening-Status and Goal Ratings on Male Adolescents

Scale		Therapist (N = 50)		Patient (N = 42)		Significant Other (N = 30)	
		Initial	Goals	Initial	Goals	Initial	Goals
Family Interaction	X̄	3.46	4.26	3.95	4.45	3.57	4.50
	sd	.68	.72	.73	.83	.90	.63
Occupation	X̄	3.14	3.92	3.14	4.26	3.40	4.37
	sd	1.24	.94	1.34	.96	1.19	.76
Getting Along with Others	X̄	3.68	4.18	4.38	4.71	3.60	4.57
	sd	1.11	.92	.96	.71	1.10	.57
Feelings and Mood	X̄	3.36	4.10	3.78	4.60	3.50	4.70
	sd	1.08	.93	1.14	.83	1.25	.60
Use of Free Time	X̄	3.40	4.00	3.71	4.40	3.53	4.63
	sd	1.03	.88	1.29	.96	1.38	.62
Problems	X̄	2.90	3.92	3.28	4.33	3.03	4.43
	sd	.84	.80	1.33	1.16	1.13	.68
Attitude toward Self	X̄	2.90	3.78	3.45	4.14	3.13	4.17
	sd	1.02	.93	1.21	1.07	1.14	.87

Table 3–15
Means and Standard Deviations for PES Opening-Status and Goal Ratings on Female Adolescents

Scale		Therapist (N = 50)		Patient (N = 41)		Significant Other (N = 21)	
		Initial	Goals	Initial	Goals	Initial	Goals
Family Interaction	$\overline{X}$	3.56	4.40	3.63	4.49	3.52	4.48
	sd	.58	.53	.80	.78	.93	.98
Occupation	$\overline{X}$	3.62	4.52	3.76	4.41	3.62	4.67
	sd	1.32	.65	1.39	.97	1.24	.66
Getting Along with Others	$\overline{X}$	3.88	4.44	4.05	4.51	3.86	4.67
	sd	.92	.64	.84	.60	1.06	.58
Feelings and Mood	$\overline{X}$	3.08	4.18	3.51	4.49	3.10	4.62
	sd	.88	.66	1.21	.87	1.44	.92
Use of Free Time	$\overline{X}$	3.22	4.14	3.39	4.39	2.95	4.10
	sd	1.15	.64	1.34	.89	1.43	1.14
Problems	$\overline{X}$	2.76	4.12	3.05	4.54	2.95	4.24
	sd	.87	.63	1.28	.78	.97	.83
Attitude toward Self	$\overline{X}$	2.78	4.00	2.90	3.90	2.67	4.20
	sd	1.00	.70	1.11	1.00	1.11	1.00

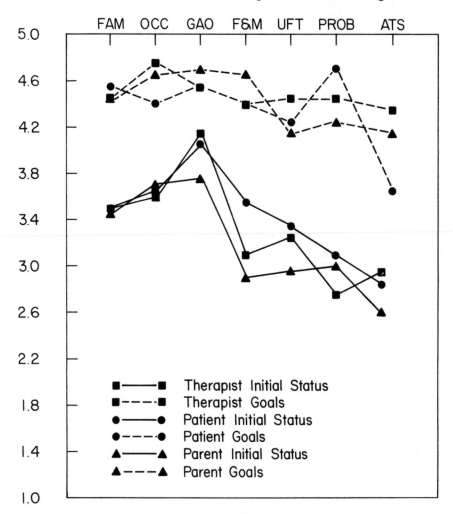

Figure 3–8. Comparison of Initial Ratings by Therapist, Patient, and Parent on Twenty Female Adolescents

status ratings are highest on several scales, whereas that of the parent is lowest. This tendency for parents of adolescents referred to a mental-health service to see their offspring as having more problems than the youngsters themselves has been reported in other studies (Gleser et al. 1980). From the current data, it appears also that parents set higher goals, on the average, than do their offspring. This could indicate that such parents tend to have unusually high expectations for their youngsters, which contributes to the youngsters' problems and to the parents' low evaluation of their behavior. Alternatively, the adolescents may set lower goals defensively in order to have a better chance of succeeding.

Correlations among therapist, patient, and significant others with respect to status and goal ratings on corresponding PES scales are shown in table 3–16 for male and table 3–17 for female adolescents. Therapists' ratings of opening status are more highly correlated with those of the adolescent than with the parents' ratings, particularly for the females. The correlations between ratings of adolescent and therapist are also higher, in general, than those between the youngsters and their parents for both sexes. The correlations among the goal ratings are different for girls than boys. The correlations between goal ratings of mother and daughter are higher than those between mother and son. Furthermore, goal ratings of the therapist show almost no agreement with those of the girls or their mothers but are correlated with the boys' goals on most scales and with those of the boys' mothers on *Family Interaction, Occupation,* and *Attitude to Self.* More research is needed to understand the reasons for these sex differences.

Means of closing-status ratings made by therapists are shown in tables 3–18 and 3–19. Comparisons with the opening-status ratings are indicated in these tables by correlations and in the figures by a comparison with goals. The adolescents, both male and female, were higher than their initial status on all scales, approaching closely the initial goals on several scales, as illustrated in figures 3–9 and 3–10. The differences were highly significant for all but the scales *Use of Free Time* for the boys and *Occupation* for the girls. Correlations between therapists' opening- and closing-status ratings are also all significant, with one or two exceptions.

An analysis of the length of treatment indicated that adolescents were seen in therapy an average of 7.8 sessions, with a range from 2 to 46. The number of sessions was significantly related to therapists' initial-status rating on two scales, with those rated as healthier seen fewer times. In particular, males seen as having a more positive *Attitude toward Self* and females who do better on *Getting Along with Others* were seen the fewest times. Those females who rated themselves high on *Feelings and Mood* also were seen relatively few times. No significant correlations were obtained between number of sessions and final status ratings.

Children: Two samples of children were analyzed for whom both parent and therapist had filled out the PES initially. The first sample consisted of 28 children. In all but 6 of these cases only the therapist had made ratings when the case was closed. Nineteen of the 28 children were male. The age range was 3 to 12 years of age, with an average of 9.1 years. The children had been seen on 1 to 8 occasions ($\overline{X} = 3.4$) over a range of from one to eight months.

Table 3–16
Correlations among PES Opening and Goal Ratings of Therapist, Patient, and Significant Other on Adolescent Males and Correlation of Ratings with Age of Adolescent

Scale	Present			Goals		
	Patient (N = 42)	Significant Other (N = 30)	Age	Patient (N = 42)	Significant Other (N = 30)	Age
Family Interaction						
Therapist	0.29	0.51	−0.11	0.17	0.49	−0.14
Patient		.45	.27		.29	.03
Significant other			.07			.16
Occupation						
Therapist	.87	.79	−.20	.66	.52	−.23
Patient		.73	−.01		.39	−.03
Significant other			−.29			.10
Getting Along with Others						
Therapist	.38	.44	−.27	.35	.24	−.19
Patient		.26	.48		.21	.40
Significant other			−.08			−.25
Feelings and Mood						
Therapist	.45	−.01	−.36	.40	.02	−.30
Patient		.22	−.08		.15	.12
Significant other			.17			.20
Use of Free Time						
Therapist	.60	.15	−.09	.45	.18	−.21
Patient		.29	.04		−.11	.06
Significant other			.21			.15
Problems						
Therapist	.46	−.03	−.28	.32	.22	−.13
Patient		.58	−.02		.07	−.01
Significant other			.14			.23
Attitude toward Self						
Therapist	.41	.63	−.17	.24	.47	−.06
Patient		.34	.23		.11	.17
Significant other			−.03			.13

Table 3–17
Correlations among PES Opening and Goal Ratings of Therapist, Patient, and Significant Other on Adolescent Females and Correlation of Ratings with Age of Adolescent

Scale	Present			Goals		
	Patient (N = 41)	Significant Other (N = 21)	Age	Patient (N = 41)	Significant Other (N = 21)	Age
Family Interaction						
Therapist	0.52	0.07	-0.25	0.10	-0.18	-0.22
Patient		.47	-.10		.21	.22
Significant other			.16			.53
Occupation						
Therapist	.85	.68	-.19	.32	-.16	-.31
Patient		.83	-.19		.69	-.08
Significant other			-.35			-.35
Getting Along with Others						
Therapist	.53	.44	.00	.12	.17	.05
Patient		.38	-.17		.41	-.17
Significant other			.20			-.12
Feelings and Mood						
Therapist	.52	.62	.02	.07	-.14	.00
Patient		.49	-.35		.58	-.04
Significant other			.11			.02
Use of Free Time						
Therapist	.58	.36	-.02	.19	.11	-.11
Patient		.42	-.24		.43	-.15
Significant other			-.29			.11
Problems						
Therapist	.63	.43	-.02	.08	-.02	-.00
Patient		.50	-.12		.31	-.03
Significant other			.22			.24
Attitude toward Self						
Therapist	.65	.38	-.00	-.02	.05	.11
Patient		.22	-.04		.22	-.04
Significant other			.20			-.34

Table 3–18

Means and Standard Deviations of PES Closing Status as Rated by Therapists and Comparison with Opening Status for Male Adolescents (N = 50)

Scale	Therapist Closing Status		Correlation between Therapist Opening and Closing Ratings	Mean Change from Therapist Opening (X̄ Closing − X̄ Opening)	t	p
	X̄	sd				
Family Interaction	3.94	0.74	0.38	0.48	4.28	<0.0001
Occupation	3.68	1.17	.51	.54	3.20	<.005
Getting Along with Others	4.12	.90	.67	.44	3.71	<.001
Feelings and Mood	3.96	1.01	.63	.60	4.71	<.0001
Use of Free Time	3.62	.90	.43	.22	1.50	ns
Problems	3.62	1.01	.41	.72	5.02	<.0001
Attitude to Self	3.70	.97	.46	.80	5.47	<.0001

Table 3–19

Means and Standard Deviations of PES Closing Status as Rated by Therapists and Comparison with Opening Status for Female Adolescents (N = 49)

Scale	Therapist Closing Status		Correlation between Therapist Opening and Closing Ratings	Mean Change from Therapist Opening (X̄ Closing − X̄ Opening)	t	p
	X̄	sd				
Family Interaction	4.10	0.65	0.34	0.54	5.39	<0.0001
Occupation	3.82	1.05	.30	.20	.99	ns
Getting Along with Others	4.41	.70	.35	.53	3.94	<.001
Feelings and Mood	3.96	.93	.44	.88	6.43	<.0001
Use of Free Time	3.71	1.02	.28	.49	2.63	<.05
Problems	3.82	.78	.17	1.06	6.97	<.0001
Attitude to Self	3.73	1.08	.43	.95	5.98	<.0001

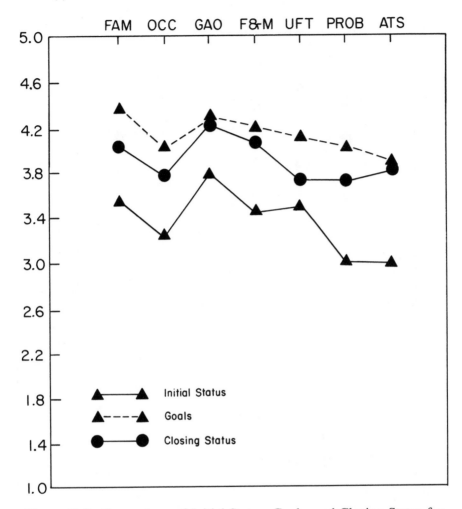

Figure 3–9. Comparison of Initial Status, Goals, and Closing Status for Fifty Outpatient Male Adolescents: Ratings by Therapists

Means and standard deviations of status ratings at opening and closing are shown in table 3–20. Both the parents and the therapists rated *Problems* and *Family Interaction* lowest initially. At closing, these were among the highest scores. The greatest improvement on *Problems* occurred with those families seen the largest number of occasions. This relationship was not found, however, for *Family Interaction,* or for any of the other scale ratings. Older children were rated higher on *Family Interaction* initially, but this relationship no longer held at closing. Therapists' ratings of school adjustment *(Occupation)* and *Getting Along with Others* were

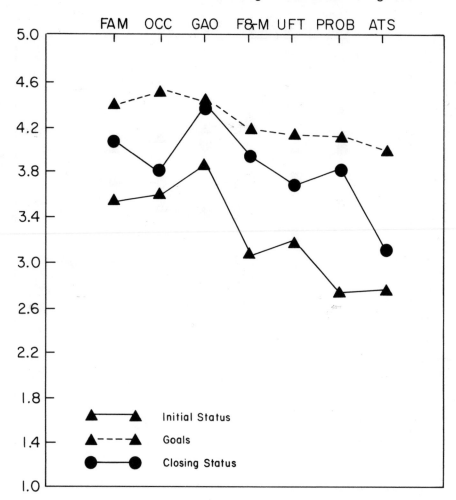

Figure 3–10. Comparison of Initial Status, Goals, and Closing Status for
Fifty Outpatient Female Adolescents: Ratings by Therapists

slightly lower at termination than initially but higher than the parents'
initial perception.

A more recently analyzed sample consisted of 50 boys and 21 girls.
The boys averaged 9.1 years of age, the girls 8.3 years. Parents' ratings
were available on 39 of the boys and 20 of the girls. Means and standard
deviations for initial status and goal ratings are shown in tables 3–21 and
3–22 and illustrated in figures 3–11 and 3–12. Differences on average
ratings between therapist and parent ranged from 0.20 to 0.38 for the

Table 3–20
Means and Standard Deviations of Initial and Closing PES Ratings on a Children's Sample (N = 28)

Scale		Opening		Closing
		Parent	*Therapist*	*Therapist*
Family Interaction	$\overline{X}$	3.11	3.39	3.86
	sd	1.29	1.34	.89
Occupation	$\overline{X}$	3.32	3.71	3.61
	sd	1.39	1.08	1.20
Getting Along with Others	$\overline{X}$	3.28	3.79	3.50
	sd	1.21	1.13	.96
Feelings and Mood	$\overline{X}$	3.69	3.38	3.59
	sd	1.28	1.24	.98
Use of Free Time	$\overline{X}$	3.55	3.69	3.79
	sd	1.09	1.00	.86
Problems	$\overline{X}$	2.86	3.34	3.62
	sd	1.38	.86	.86

boys and from 0.00 to 0.63 for the girls. This largest mean difference occurs for *Getting Along with Others*. The difference of 0.56 between means for *Family Interaction* is also sizable. The low ratings on *Family Interaction* and *Getting Along with Others* suggest that the mothers were particularly concerned about their daughters' socialization. As noted with

Table 3–21
Means and Standard Deviations for PES Opening-Status Ratings on Male and Female Children by Therapist and Parent

Scale		Therapist		Parent	
		Male (N = 50)	*Female* (N = 21)	*Male* (N = 39)	*Female* (N = 20)
Family Interaction	$\overline{X}$	3.54	3.76	3.28	3.20
	sd	.81	.94	.86	.89
Occupation	$\overline{X}$	3.88	4.14	4.08	4.00
	sd	1.04	.85	1.08	1.08
Getting Along with Others	$\overline{X}$	3.46	3.43	3.18	2.80
	sd	1.05	.92	1.05	.62
Feelings and Mood	$\overline{X}$	3.26	2.95	3.46	3.00
	sd	1.06	.97	1.17	1.34
Use of Free Time	$\overline{X}$	3.66	3.05	3.28	2.90
	sd	.94	.80	1.26	1.33
Problems	$\overline{X}$	3.18	3.05	3.44	3.15
	sd	.75	.86	.99	1.04
Attitude toward Self	$\overline{X}$	2.96[a]	2.90	2.66[b]	2.90
	sd	.89	.89	.85	1.02

[a]N = 49.
[b]N = 38.

Table 3–22
Means and Standard Deviations for PES Opening-Goal Ratings on
Male and Female Children by Therapist and Parent

Scale		Therapist		Parent	
		Male (N = 50)	Female (N = 21)	Male (N = 39)	Female (N = 20)
Family Interaction	$\overline{X}$	4.28	4.38	4.20	4.10
	sd	.67	.80	.70	1.16
Occupation	$\overline{X}$	4.38	4.67	4.69	4.70
	sd	.78	.48	.52	.47
Getting Along with Others	$\overline{X}$	4.06	4.19	4.46	4.30
	sd	.87	.60	.64	.66
Feelings and Mood	$\overline{X}$	4.08	4.05	4.69	4.70
	sd	.94	.74	.57	.66
Use of Free Time	$\overline{X}$	4.22	4.10	4.44	4.35
	sd	.79	.77	.82	.81
Problems	$\overline{X}$	4.16	3.95	4.49	4.50
	sd	.76	.67	.56	.51
Attitude toward Self	$\overline{X}$	3.90[a]	3.67	4.10[b]	4.20
	sd	.87	.91	.80	.77

[a]N = 49.
[b]N = 38.

adolescents, the parents' goals for both boys and girls are considerably higher on most scales than are those of the therapists. There is very little difference between the opening status of boys and girls as rated by the therapist. Only the difference on *Use of Free Time* is significant ($p<0.05$). Here boys score higher than girls. None of the parents' ratings differ significantly.

Correlations between ratings of parent and therapist are presented in tables 3–23 and 3–24. The correlations between initial-status ratings for boys range from 0.07 to 0.79, with a median of 0.40. For the girls, the range is from 0.06 to 0.82, and the median correlation is 0.22. The correlations between the two sets of goal ratings are modest, with a median of 0.38 for the boys and 0.32 for the girls. Age is related principally to *Family Interaction*.

Tables 3–25 and 3–26 contain the mean closing-status ratings of the therapist and a comparison between these and the opening-status ratings. Both boys and girls have moved nearer to the goals set by the therapist (see table 3–22). They differ from each other very little with respect to their outcome scores except that the boys now have a significantly higher mean score on *Attitude toward Self*. The difference in *Use of Free Time* noted initially is still apparent but no longer significant. Improvement was highly significant statistically on all scales except *Occupation* and *Use of Free Time* for the boys. Considerably less improvement was noted

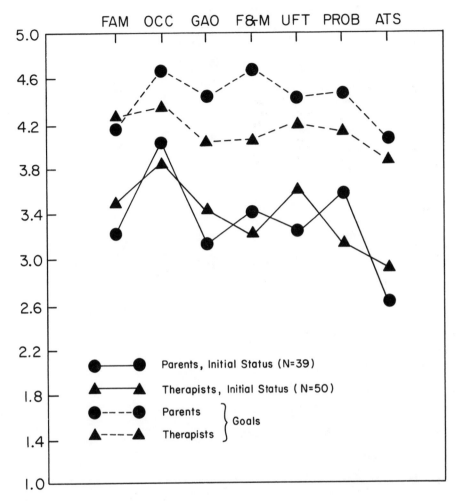

Figure 3–11. Comparison of Ratings by Parents and Therapists for Outpatient Male Children

for the girls, with only the ratings for *Feelings and Mood* reaching the
0.05 level of significance. More research is needed to understand the
reasons for this sex difference.

The children (or the family) were seen an average of 7.8 times.
Number of sessions was significantly positively correlated with therapists'
closing-status ratings on *Family Interaction, Feelings and Mood,* and
Attitude toward Self for boys but not for girls. Only mothers' opening-
status rating of *Feelings and Mood* and therapists' opening ratings of *Use*

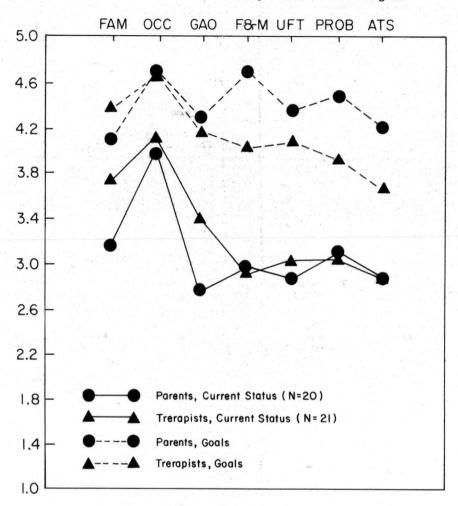

Figure 3–12. Comparison of Ratings by Parents and Therapists for Outpatient Female Children

of Free Time were significantly correlated with number of sessions for
girls, with both correlations indicating a negative relationship.

One possible reason for the general lack of relationship found between
number of sessions and outcome for both children and adolescents is the
fact that only sessions that actually involved the youngster were counted.
Thus, in some cases, therapeutic gains may have been accomplished by
seeing the parents, but unless the children also were present, these sessions
were not part of the total number of sessions for each child. Thus a child

Table 3–23
Correlations between Therapist and Parent PES Opening-Status and Goal Ratings on Male Children and Correlations between Ratings and Age of Child

Scale	Present		Goals	
	Parent (N = 39)	Age	Parent (N = 39)	Age
Family Interaction				
Therapist	0.40	0.23	0.55	0.01
Parent		.52		.23
Occupation				
Therapist	.79	.03	.44	−.02
Parent		.04		.04
Getting Along with Others				
Therapist	.48	.18	.38	−.05
Parent		−.03		.08
Feelings and Mood				
Therapist	.23	.20	.28	−.02
Parent		−.05		−.23
Use of Free Time				
Therapist	.32	.08	.41	−.03
Parent		.05		−.12
Problems				
Therapist	.40	−.15	.30	−.20
Parent		.23		−.07
Attitude toward Self				
Therapist	.07	.12	−.08	−.07
Parent		−.14		−.21

could improve considerably without having been seen more than two or three times individually. Further research is needed to explore the relationship of the total number of sessions a family is seen and the treatment outcome of the child.

Conclusion

The median reliability of therapists' status and goal ratings for children and adolescents on the PES is estimated to be about 0.44. This coefficient is an intraclass correlation, which takes into account differences in mean ratings of therapist. The average error variance for ratings is approximately 0.36, yielding a standard error of measurement of 0.6. This implies that 95 percent of the time, ratings on any one scale would be fewer than 1.2 points from that obtainable if a large number of ratings were made on a child at the same point in time.

Ratings of current status on the PES sharply distinguish groups of normal children from those seen in a community mental-health center or

Table 3–24

Correlation between Therapist and Parent PES Opening-Status and Goal Ratings on Female Children and Correlation between Ratings and Age of Child

	Present		Goals	
Scale	Parent (N = 20)	Age	Parent (N = 20)	Age
Family Interaction				
Therapist	0.61	0.65	0.51	0.64
Parent		.79		.69
Occupation				
Therapist	.82	.18	.76	− .02
Parent		.19		.15
Getting Along with Others				
Therapist	.19	− .05	.22	.23
Parent		.35		.17
Feelings and Mood				
Therapist	.16	− .26	.29	− .02
Parent		.25		.25
Use of Free Time				
Therapist	.06	− .21	.17	.01
Parent		.22		.17
Problems				
Therapist	.22	− .08	.32	.07
Parent		.28		.12
Attitude toward Self				
Therapist	.34	− .13	.32	− .05
Parent		− .12		− .23

classes for the emotionally impaired. All three groups are distinguished from children enrolled in a partial-hospitalization program. A similar differentiation also occurs for groups of male and female adolescents.

Status ratings on the seven PES scales are only modestly intercorrelated in normative samples. Average intercorrelations obtained were 0.30 for adolescent girls, 0.16 for adolescent boys, and 0.22 for a mixed sample.

Initial status as rated by therapist, adolescent, and significant other are substantially intercorrelated on most scales. Goal ratings are much less well correlated, particularly for adolescent females. Correlations between status and goal ratings of therapist and parent for children vary considerably from one scale to another and are inconsistent for the sexes.

The PES scales were shown to correlate moderately and meaningfully with two other self-report measures for a sample of normal adolescents.

The PES scales demonstrate sensitivity to change in status. Ratings at termination of therapy increased significantly over initial-status scores on samples of male and female adolescents and on a sample of male

Table 3–25

Means and Standard Deviations of PES Closing Status as Rated by Therapists and Comparison with Opening Status for Male Children (N = 50)

Scale	Therapist Closing Status		Correlation between Therapist Opening and Closing Ratings	Mean Change from Therapist Opening ($\bar{X}$ Closing − $\bar{X}$ Opening)	t	p
	$\bar{X}$	sd				
Family Interaction	3.96	0.83	0.52	0.42	3.70	0.001
Occupation	4.06	.93	.51	.18	1.30	ns
Getting Along with Others	3.92	.92	.35	.46	2.88	.01
Feelings and Mood	3.74	1.05	.37	.48	2.87	.01
Use of Free Time	3.78	1.00	.59	.12	.96	ns
Problems	3.74	.90	.28	.56	3.97	.001
Attitude toward Self	3.68	1.02	.40	.72	4.79	.001

Table 3–26

Means and Standard Deviations of PES Closing Status as Rated by Therapists and Comparison with Opening Status for Female Children (N = 21)

Scale	Therapist Closing Status		Correlation between Therapist Opening and Closing Ratings	Mean Change from Therapist Opening ($\bar{X}$ Closing − $\bar{X}$ Opening)	t	p
	$\bar{X}$	sd				
Family Interaction	4.00	0.77	0.34	0.24	1.11	ns
Occupation	4.45	.76	.18	.31	1.34	ns
Getting Along with Others	3.57	.87	.74	.14	.99	ns
Feelings and Mood	3.57	1.16	.51	.62	2.66	.05
Use of Free Time	3.38	.86	.26	.33	1.50	ns
Problems	3.52	.81	.18	.47	2.01	.06
Attitude toward Self	3.05	1.16	.15	.15	.51	ns

children. Similar increases were obtained for a small group of female children, but the changes failed to reach significance on most scales, probably due to the small size of the sample. Number of therapy sessions is not related to outcome for adolescent and children samples.

4

Application of Progress Evaluation Scales to Developmentally Disabled Populations

Generalizability Studies

In an early stage of the development of the Progress Evaluation Scales, a study was undertaken to investigate the extent of agreement between raters in their use of the scales with developmentally disabled clients. Only the first six scales were used since the seventh scale, *Attitude toward Self,* had not yet been constructed.

Ratings were obtained on two samples, each of 20 developmentally disabled clients: an institutionalized group and a group living in the community and attending a sheltered workshop. The institutionalized sample was rated independently by two aides; the community sample by an aide and her supervisor, both of whom worked directly with the clients. In each sample all ratings were made by the same two persons. In both cases, the raters had had no prior experience with the PES.

The mean ratings of current status and goals on the PES for both samples are presented in table 4–1. An analysis of variance of the two sets of ratings for each sample yielded estimates of variance for "true" score ($\hat{\sigma}_p^2$), error ($\hat{\sigma}_e^2$), and expected observed score ($\hat{\sigma}_x^2$) of current status and goals. These estimates are also contained in table 4–1. The ratio of $\hat{\sigma}_p^2$ to $\hat{\sigma}_x^2$ is an intraclass correlation, r_{xx}, which is a measure of the expected reliability of a qualified rater in using the scales, assuming the same rater assesses all clients. These coefficients (termed *generalizability coefficients*) are shown in table 4–1.

The table shows that the community clients were rated somewhat higher on most scales than were the institutionalized. They were also a much more homogeneous group as indicated by the smaller estimates of observed score variance. For both groups, the goals were set very close to the status ratings, indicating that for these clients little more is expected than to maintain the current level of functioning.

Mean differences in ratings were rather large on *Family Interaction* and *Problems* for the community clients and on *Getting Along with Others* for the institutionalized. However, the error variances for all scales save *Problems* were not much larger than those obtained with mental-health-center clients, ranging from 0.08 to 0.75. The generalizability coefficients were reasonably high for ratings on the institutionalized clients, averaging 0.74 for current status and 0.75 for goals. They were somewhat lower

Table 4–1
Comparison of Ratings on Two Developmentally Disabled Adult Samples of Twenty Clients Each

Scale	Present Rating						Goal (Six Months)					
	M_{t_1}	M_{t_2}	$\hat{\sigma}^2_x$	$\hat{\sigma}^2_p$	$\hat{\sigma}^2_e$	r_{xx}	M_{t_1}	M_{t_2}	$\hat{\sigma}^2_x$	$\hat{\sigma}^2_p$	$\hat{\sigma}^2_e$	r_{xx}
Community clients												
Family Interaction	3.10	3.60	0.70	0.25	0.45	0.36	3.55	4.25	0.61	0.16	0.45	0.26
Occupation	4.30	4.00	.44	.14	.30	.32	4.30	3.95	.42	.10	.32	.24
Getting Along with Others	3.75	3.55	.34	.24	.10	.71	3.85	3.55	.39	.21	.18	.54
Feelings and Mood	3.90	4.10	.99	.44	.55	.44	4.05	4.10	.80	.42	.38	.53
Use of Free Time	2.90	2.85	.80	.62	.18	.77	3.10	3.10	.72	.42	.30	.58
Problems	2.40	3.70	1.10	0	1.10	0	2.45	3.60	1.06	.04	1.02	.04
Institutionalized Clients												
Family Interaction	2.50	2.50	1.42	1.27	.15	.89	2.65	2.75	1.52	1.40	.12	.92
Occupation	2.15	2.00	1.60	1.52	.08	.95	2.25	2.15	1.85	1.75	.10	.95
Getting Along with Others	2.95	2.00	1.12	.69	.42	.62	3.15	3.20	1.19	.87	.32	.73
Feelings and Mood	3.85	3.45	1.64	.89	.75	.54	4.05	3.70	1.05	.52	.52	.50
Use of Free Time	2.20	2.30	1.74	1.19	.55	.68	2.30	2.60	1.95	1.30	.65	.67
Problems	3.80	3.65	3.19	2.51	.68	.79	3.95	3.90	2.54	1.92	.62	.75

for the ratings on community clients, partly because of the greater homogeneity of that group.

After obtaining these results, inquiries were made regarding the difficulty noted with respect to the scale for *Problems* with the community clients. It was found that one of the staff was rating the developmental disability as a problem, hence lowering her ratings. As a result of our inquiry, use of this scale was clarified.

More recently a second study of rater reliability was undertaken using all seven scales of the PES. For this study, 61 developmentally disabled clients institutionalized at the Oakdale Regional Center for the Developmental Disabilities in Michigan were evaluated by the case manager and the aide assigned to them after a two-hour training session.[a] These clients ranged from moderately to profoundly developmentally disabled, thus providing scores ranging from 1 to 5 on all but *Family Interaction* where the highest score was 4.

As indicated in table 4–2, the mean ratings of case manager and aide differed significantly on all current-status ratings except *Family Interaction* and *Getting Along with Others*. They also differed significantly on four of the seven mean goal ratings. Differences in mean score profile are portrayed in figures 4–1 and 4–2. These differences yield the estimates of variance shown in the column of table 4–2 labeled $\hat{\sigma}_r^2$. The residual error variance is displayed in the next column ($\hat{\sigma}_e^2$). The mean differences contribute to error only if case managers and aides are used interchangeably to evaluate clients. This probably would not be the case in most studies. However, case managers or aides will usually differ in identity from one client to another, according to who has contact with that individual, as was true in this sample. Such differences among raters increase the apparent difference among clients by inflating $\hat{\sigma}_p^2$, which should reflect only true differences between clients. We have attempted to estimate $\hat{\sigma}_p^2$ by removing $\hat{\sigma}_r^2$, but our estimates may be too small if case managers or aides differ less among themselves than case managers differ from aides in their mean ratings.

The error variances are considerably larger than those found in the previous sample where the same aide and case manager were used for all clients. Estimates of error variance range from 0.39 to 1.10 for current status and 0.39 to 0.88 for goals with a median of 0.69 and 0.67 respectively. This implies that 90 percent of all ratings in current status would be between 1.0 and 1.73 units from that which would be obtained if a very large number of evaluators were to make the same rating on that client. The 90 percent confidence interval for goals would range from

[a]Thanks are extended to David Ethridge, superintendent of the facility, for providing all the necessary assistance with this data collection.

Table 4–2
Reliability of Ratings on a Sample of Developmentally Disabled Institutionalized Adults (N = 61)

Scale	Means		σ_x^2	σ_p^2	σ_r^2	σ_e^2	r_{xx}
	Case Manager	Aide					
Current-status ratings							
Family Interaction	2.31	2.48	1.26	0.87	0.01	0.39	0.69
Occupation	3.56**	3.00**	1.85	1.05	.16	.80	.57
Getting Along with Others	3.07	3.25	1.93	1.12	.01	.81	.58
Feelings and Mood	4.00*	3.69*	1.59	.99	.05	.60	.62
Use of Free Time	3.21**	2.57**	1.35	.28	.21	1.10	.20
Problems	3.82**	3.51*	1.98	1.29	.05	.69	.65
Attitude toward Self	3.51**	4.00**	1.34	.81	.12	.53	.60
Goal ratings							
Family Interaction	2.82	2.97	1.84	1.38	.02	.46	.75
Occupation	3.98**	3.38**	1.56	.85	.18	.71	.54
Getting Along with Others	3.49	3.59	1.87	.99	0	.88	.53
Feelings and Mood	4.15	4.08	1.61	1.12	0	.49	.70
Use of Free Time	3.69**	3.10**	1.32	.53	.18	.79	.40
Problems	4.17*	3.77*	1.67	1.00	.08	.67	.60
Attitude toward Self	3.82**	4.21**	1.12	.73	.08	.39	.65

$*p < 0.05.$
$**p < 0.01.$

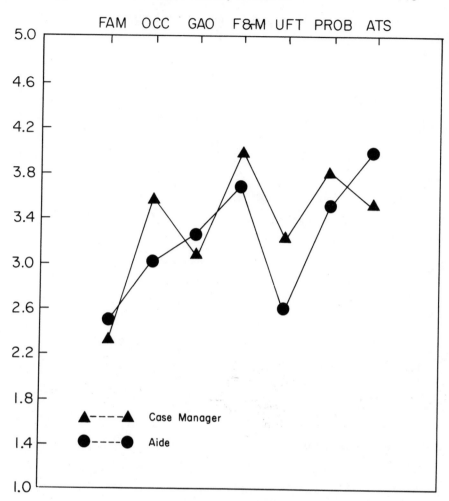

Figure 4–1. Comparison of Initial-Status Ratings by Case Manager and
Aide for Institutionalized Developmentally Disabled Clients
(N = 61)

1.0 to 1.55. The rather poor precision found in this study could be due
to a number of factors. One is that the case manager and the aide see the
client under different circumstances, thus getting a somewhat different
perspective of his or her functioning. If this is the case, it might be better
to obtain ratings from both and average them to obtain greater generalizability. Averaging would yield a score having only half the error variance of the separate scores. Another possibility is that the client's behavior
varies from morning to evening so that aides on different shifts use

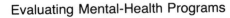

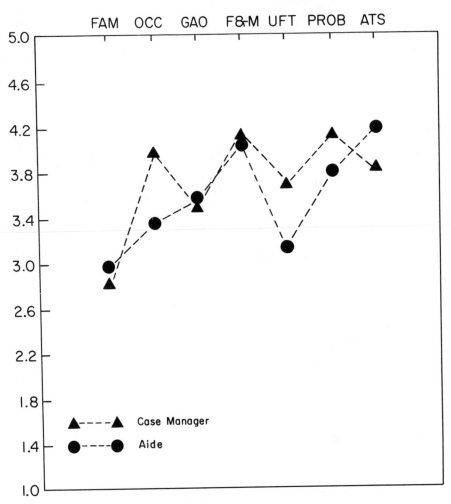

Figure 4–2. Comparison of Six-Month Goal Ratings by Case Manager and Aide for Institutionalized Developmentally Disabled Clients (N = 61)

different information for their ratings. Here, again, an average of ratings made over a day would reduce error. The third possibility is that the scales are interpreted differently by different evaluators, in which case more training would increase precision.

The reliability coefficients in the last column were computed under the assumption that either one case manager or one aide would make ratings on all clients in future use with this scale. The intent, however, is to generalize to the average rating of a large number of such evaluators whose average scores would reflect observations of the client in many situations throughout the day. These coefficients range from 0.20 to 0.69 for current status, with a median of 0.60, and from 0.40 to 0.75 for goals, with a median of .060.

Construct Validity Studies

Comparison among Developmentally Disabled Groups

The 61 institutionalized developmentally disabled in the sample were divided into three subgroups on the basis of their IQ scores or other pertinent criteria of intellectual functioning. These subgroups consisted of 16 moderately disabled females, 15 severely disabled males, and a mixed group of 30 profoundly disabled males and females. The ratings of case manager and aide were averaged for these subgroups; the resulting values are presented in table 4–3. The current status and goal ratings are also compared in figures 4–3 and 4–4.

The three groups differed significantly ($p < .01$ or better) and in the expected order on current status on all scales with the exception of *Use of Free Time* by an analysis of variance. For this scale, also, the difference between the profoundly disabled group and the moderately disabled is significant ($p \leq 0.05$), with the mean for the severely disabled falling halfway in between. The main differentiations between the moderate and severe groups are in the areas of *Family Interaction* and *Occupation*. These differences are suspect, however, since they could be partially attributable to sex differences rather than severity of disability. This is particularly likely for *Family Interaction*, judging from other data we have examined. All scales except *Use of Free Time* differentiate the profoundly disabled from each of the other two groups.

The goals for the three groups differ significantly and even more markedly than does current status, as can be seen clearly in figure 4–4. Goals for the moderately disabled are set higher than for the other two groups relative to their initial status, thus separating them from the goals for the severely disabled. (This tendency was not noted for groups differing only by sex.)

An additional sample, 62 developmentally disabled male and female clients currently enrolled in community mental-health programs (supervised work activity and a sheltered workshop), was evaluated. They were diagnosed as mildly and moderately disabled. Their average current status

Table 4–3
Means and Standard Deviations of Combined PES Ratings on Samples of Developmentally Disabled, Classified by Severity

Scale	Moderate (Females, N = 16)				Severe (Males, N = 15)				Profound (Males and Females, N = 30)			
	Status		Goals		Status		Goals		Status		Goals	
	X̄	sd	X̄	sd	X̄	sd	X̄	sd	X̄	sd	X̄	sd
Family Interaction	3.35	.57	4.22	.54	2.64	.85	3.36	.81	1.77	.89	1.95	.94
Occupation	4.09	1.23	4.69	.57	3.57	1.19	4.13	.95	2.70	1.05	2.92	1.00
Getting Along with Others	3.97	1.13	4.52	.85	3.70	1.10	4.10	1.05	2.45	.94	2.76	.88
Feelings and Mood	4.32	.79	4.78	.36	4.40	.91	4.66	.59	3.36	1.18	3.56	1.08
Use of Free Time	3.34	1.13	4.31	.79	2.96	1.03	3.73	.90	2.62	.91	2.73	.81
Problems	4.32	.77	4.78	.36	4.34	1.13	4.46	1.01	2.98	1.28	3.28	1.19
Attitude toward Self	4.47	.65	4.81	.25	4.20	.92	4.46	.83	3.15	1.04	3.36	.93

Note: "Combined" refers to average of ratings by case manager and aide. All ratings except *Use of Free Time* status ratings differ significantly among the three groups.

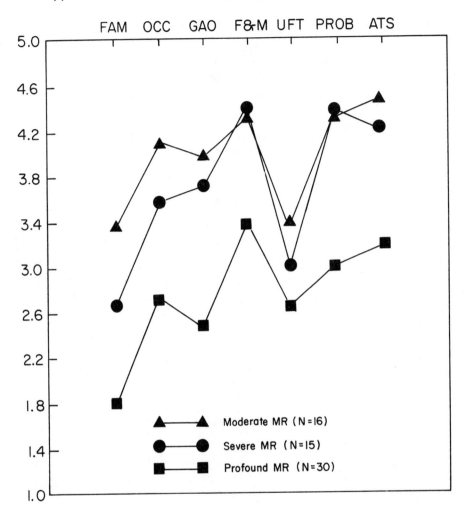

Figure 4–3. Comparison on Current-Status Functioning among Three
   Groups of Developmentally Disabled, Classified by Severity

and goal ratings are presented in table 4–4 and illustrated in figure 4–5.
The ratings were made by the unit manager of the ACKCO day program
in Shiawassee County, Michigan, who supervises part of the work activities and sheltered workshop programs.
   Comparing figure 4–5 with figure 4–6, which shows the moderately
disabled institutionalized sample, a number of differences can be noted.
The community group is higher on *Occupation* than the institutionalized

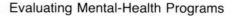

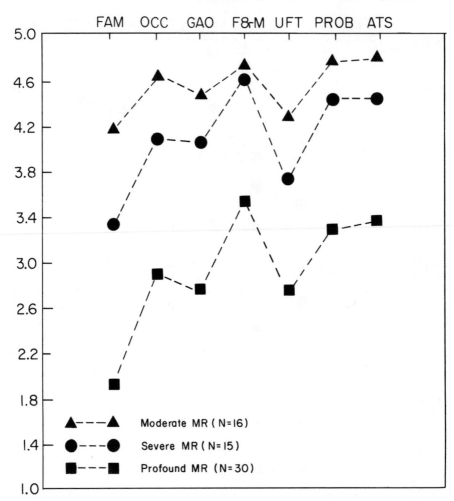

Figure 4–4. Comparison of Goals Set by Supervisors for Three Groups
of Institutionalized Developmentally Disabled Clients

but lower on the next five scales and very significantly lower on *Feelings and Mood* ($p < 0.01$), *Problems* ($p < 0.001$) and *Attitude toward Self* ($p < 0.001$). *Use of Free Time* is also significantly lower ($p = 0.05$). One can only speculate on what these differences mean. One possibility is that the scales are being interpreted differently in the two settings. This may account for some differences but seems unlikely to account for the large differences, for instance, in *Feelings and Mood* and *Attitude toward Self*. Differences in available occupational and recreational opportunities might

Table 4–4
Means, Standard Deviations, and Correlations for Two Samples of Developmentally Disabled Clients for Current Functioning and Goals

Scale	Mild and Moderate[a] (N = 62)			Infirm (N = 33)		
	Present	Goals	r_{pg}	Present	Goals	r_{pg}
Family Interaction						
$\overline{X}$	3.39	3.56	0.94	1.12	1.24	0.45
sd	1.15	1.03		.42	.50	
Occupation						
$\overline{X}$	4.56	4.66	.95	2.27	2.91	.17
sd	.92	.79		.63	.52	
Getting Along with Others						
$\overline{X}$	3.63	3.89	.86	3.61	4.30	.54
sd	1.01	.87		.83	.82	
Feelings and Mood						
$\overline{X}$	3.61	3.85	.93	3.70	4.21	.29
sd	1.16	.97		1.02	.86	
Use of Free Time						
$\overline{X}$	2.66	2.89	.93	2.09	3.58	-.11
sd	1.28	1.37		1.13	.66	
Problems						
$\overline{X}$	3.42	3.60	.94	3.39	4.52	-.32
sd	1.12	1.08		.83	.67	
Attitude toward Self						
$\overline{X}$	3.00	3.23	.93	3.00	3.27	.37
sd	1.16	1.08		.66	.52	

[a]Enrolled in community programs.

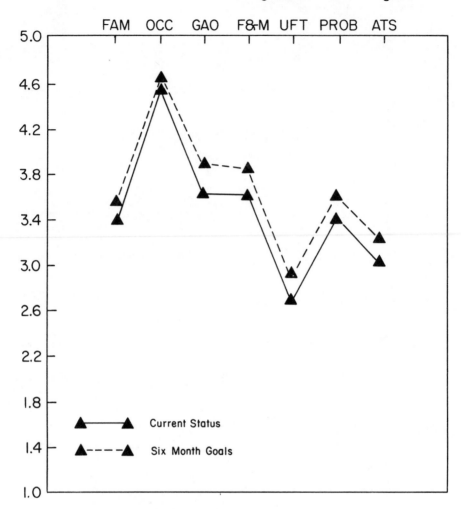

Figure 4–5. Current Status and Goals for Developmentally Disabled
Clients Enrolled in Community Programs (N = 62)

account for the difference on *Occupation* and *Use of Free Time*. The
large differences on *Problems, Feelings and Mood* and *Attitude toward
Self,* however, seem likely to reflect the difficulty for the developmentally
disabled in adapting to community life and trying to meet at least some
of its standards.

It may also be noted from figures 4–5 and 4–6 that higher six-month
goals were set for the institutionalized clients relative to their current
status than were those for the community clients. The simplest explanation

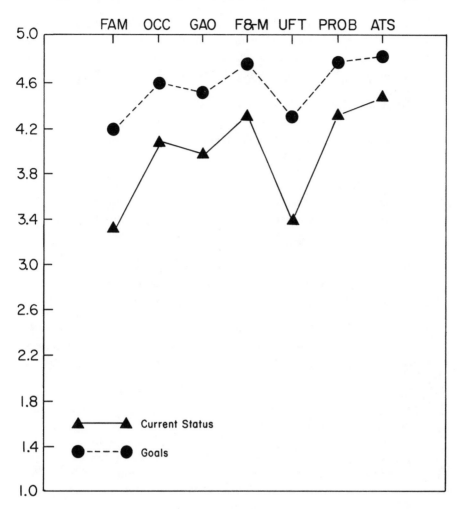

Figure 4–6. Comparison of Current Status and Goals for Institutionalized
Moderate Developmentally Disabled Clients (N = 16)

for this is that raters in the institution had no experience with these scales
before and therefore little idea of what constituted reasonably obtainable
goals on these dimensions. In this regard, the correlations between current
status and six-month goal ratings shown in the third column of table 4–4
indicate that the goals set by the community case manager are almost
entirely determined by his perception of current status. A comparison
with the last column, which relates current status to goals in another
sample, indicates that such goal setting is not necessarily so determined.

These data pertain to a group of males and females rated in the infirmary of the Oakdale Institution. They are a mixed group of chronically and acutely ill clients. Evidently the goals in this case are more dependent on the physical status of the patient and the chronicity of his or her illness.

Sex Difference and Correlations with Age and IQ

Samples of 39 male and 36 female developmentally disabled who were living in Shiawassee County and whose age and IQ were known were rated on the PES by their case managers. The males averaged 32.3 years, with a standard deviation of 13.7, whereas the women averaged 40.8 years, with a standard deviation of 14.4. The difference in age is significant ($p \leq 0.05$). Their average IQs (56.3) were almost identical, although there was a wider range of scores for the males (sd = 19.2) than the females (13.5).

The means and standard deviations of PES current-status ratings and the correlations with age and IQ are shown in table 4–5 for each sex separately. Females were rated significantly higher than males on *Family Interaction* and *Use of Free Time*. All other mean differences were very small; standard deviations were similar as well. Only the scale *Family Interaction* correlated significantly with IQ, and this relationship was found to be present for both sexes. Those men and women having higher IQs were rated higher on *Family Interaction*. In addition, older women were rated higher than younger women on *Family Interaction* ($r = 0.40$), but this relationship did not hold for men. The correlations between age and IQ were negligible in both samples.

Goal ratings for these two samples and correlations with age and IQ are shown in table 4–6. There are no significant sex differences in these means, nor do the standard deviations differ significantly. *Family Interaction* is, again, significantly correlated with age for the females and with IQ for both sexes. However, for goal ratings, *Occupation* is significantly negatively correlated with age in both samples, as is *Feelings and Mood* for the female sample. That is, older men and women are not expected to do as well with regard to occupational adjustment as the younger clients, and older women are expected to have less control of feelings and moods than are younger women. For men, both *Family Interaction* and *Occupational* adjustment are expected to improve more for those with higher IQ.

Intercorrelations among PES Scale Ratings

Intercorrelations among case managers' PES scale ratings were obtained for each sex separately and are shown in table 4–7 for current status and

Table 4–5
Means and Standard Deviations of Case Managers' PES Current-Status Ratings and Correlations with Age and IQ

| | Males (N = 39) | | | | Females (N = 36) | | | |
| | | | Correlations | | | | Correlations | |
	$\bar{X}$	sd	Age	IQ	$\bar{X}$	sd	Age	IQ
IQ	56.33	19.22			56.25	13.54		0.14
Age	32.36[a]	13.70		-0.27	40.75[a]	14.44		.39[b]
Family Interaction	3.18[a]	1.19	-0.08	.40[b]	3.92[a]	1.00	0.40[b]	.01
Occupation	3.38	1.82	-.23	-.07	3.28	1.85	-.29	.05
Getting Along with Others	3.82	.72	-.13	.22	3.89	.82	-.23	.05
Feelings and Mood	4.00	.89	-.14	-.06	3.92	.81	-.10	-.04
Use of Free Time	2.33[a]	1.11	-.20	.10	3.00[a]	1.12	-.04	.05
Problems	3.79	.92	-.03	-.26	3.94	.92	.20	.05
Attitude toward Self	3.59	.99	-.10	-.07	3.44	1.00	.20	-.26

[a]Means differ significantly, $p \leq 0.01$.
[b]Significant correlations, $p \leq 0.05$.

Table 4–6
Means and Standard Deviations of Case Managers' PES Goal Ratings and Correlations with Age and IQ

| | Males (N = 39) | | | | Females (N = 36) | | | |
| | | | Correlations | | | | Correlations | |
Scale	$\bar{X}$	sd	Age	IQ	$\bar{X}$	sd	Age	IQ
Family Interaction	3.62	1.07	-0.10	0.50[a]	3.92	0.94	0.40[a]	.40[a]
Occupation	4.56	1.02	-.40[a]	.43[a]	4.11	1.37	-.39[a]	.11
Getting Along with Others	4.08	.66	.06	.26	4.14	.80	-.28	-.06
Feelings and Mood	4.49	.64	-.08	.14	4.25	.69	-.38[a]	-.05
Use of Free Time	3.18	.97	.09	.21	3.31	.92	-.04	-.09
Problems	4.33	.74	.16	-.05	4.31	.79	-.03	.17
Attitude toward Self	4.15	.78	.01	.10	3.94	.86	-.04	.00

[a]Significant correlations, $p \leq 0.05$.

Table 4–7
Intercorrelations among Case Managers' PES Ratings of Developmentally Disabled Clients

Scale	Male (N = 39)						Female (N = 36)					
	2	3	4	5	6	7	2	3	4	5	6	7
Current Status												
1 Family Interaction	0.48	0.35	0.05	0.41	0.06	0.04	0.35	0.27	0.11	0.41	0.20	0.07
2 Occupation		.30	.21	.42	.30	.12		.27	.02	.55	.21	.13
3 Getting Along with Others			.45	.18	.38	.34			.55	.47	.56	.31
4 Feelings and Mood				.51	.61	.60				.44	.68	.51
5 Use of Free Time					.33	.46					.47	.54
6 Problems						.58						.62
7 Attitude toward Self												
Goals												
1 Family Interaction	.28	.15	.13	.40	−.04	−.14	.21	.05	.16	.16	.20	.03
2 Occupation		.24	.33	.19	.20	.12		.30	.33	.15	.37	.08
3 Getting Along with Others			.34	.22	.38	.38			.50	.41	.57	.34
4 Feelings and Mood				.53	.65	.59				.42	.60	.55
5 Use of Free Time					.21	.30					.42	.42
6 Problems						.50						.57
7 Attitude toward Self												

for goals. The intercorrelations of current status appear quite similar for males and females, ranging from 0.04 to 0.61 for males and 0.02 to 0.68 for females. In no case do the correlations differ significantly. The pattern of intercorrelations is also similar to that obtained for other adult clients, except that *Use of Free Time* in the present status samples is more highly correlated with *Family Interaction* and *Occupation*. Two factors account for these intercorrelations. Factor 1 is loaded on scores 1, 2, and 5 and probably represents an "everyday routine" factor, while factor 2 has loadings on scales 3, 4, 6, and 7 and might be termed an "affect" factor.

The intercorrelations among goal ratings are also not different for males as compared to females, ranging from -0.14 to 0.65 for males and 0.03 to 0.60 for females. These correlations are somewhat lower than those obtained for goal ratings of other adult clients, indicating that goals on the various scales are made less globally. Such variables as age and intellectual capacity apparently are taken into consideration by staff in making goal ratings.

Comparison of PES Ratings of Case Managers with Those of Significant Others

Among the developmentally disabled clients residing in Shiawassee County, Michigan, in 1979, there were 38 males and 36 females who had been rated by their case managers and also by a parent or guardian. The means and standard deviations for these ratings of current status are compared in tables 4–8 and 4–9 for males and females, respectively. Correlations between ratings of case manager and significant other are also displayed. Similar information for goal ratings is shown in tables 4–10 and 4–11.

The mean current-status ratings in tables 4–8 and 4–9 show that case managers' ratings are slightly lower than those of significant others on most scales for both males and females, but this difference is significant only for ratings of *Use of Free Time*. Correlations between ratings on the same scale are italicized in the tables. These values are quite high, ranging from 0.56 to 0.92 for males, with a median of 0.70, and 0.35 to 0.82 for females, with a median of 0.56. For both samples the highest correlations are for scales 1, 2, and 5, which we have identified as scales loading on a "daily routine" factor. However, each of these scales shows valid specific variance since the correlations between ratings of therapist and significant other on these scales are higher than those between ratings on different scales. The correlations between ratings of therapist and significant other on *Getting Along with Others* and *Feelings and Mood* are also higher than those for noncorresponding scales in both samples.

Table 4–8
Correlations between Current-Status Ratings of Significant Others and Case Managers for Developmentally Disabled Males (N = 38)

Significant Others	X̄	sd	Case Managers						
			1	2	3	4	5	6	7
X̄			2.68	3.26	3.66	4.24	2.26[a]	3.92	3.61
sd			1.21	1.94	.94	.79	1.11	1.02	.95
1 Family Interaction	2.74	1.31	.92	.41	.28	.11	.65	.23	.28
2 Occupation	3.39	1.85	.42	.86	.27	.14	.46	.33	.40
3 Getting Along with Others	3.89	1.01	.28	−.18	.62	.48	.22	.52	.35
4 Feelings and Mood	4.24	1.13	.14	.24	.33	.70	.30	.44	.60
5 Use of Free Time	2.66[a]	1.46	.58	.48	.29	.21	.73	.36	.39
6 Problems	3.79	1.23	.37	.19	.38	.64	.28	.56	.62
7 Attitude toward Self	3.82	1.11	.22	.32	.35	.36	.37	.56	.67

Note: Correlations between ratings on the same scale are italicized.
[a]Means differ significantly, $p \leq 0.05$.

Table 4–9
Correlations between Current-Status Ratings of Significant Others and Case Managers for Developmentally Disabled Females (N = 36)

Significant Others	X̄	sd	Case Managers						
			1	2	3	4	5	6	7
X̄			3.33	3.00	3.83	4.08	2.67[a]	3.92	3.61
sd			1.31	1.88	.81	.84	1.35	.94	1.08
1 Family Interaction	3.56	1.25	.82	−.01	.49	.28	.55	.50	.38
2 Occupation	3.42	1.57	.32	.68	.28	−.11	.47	.16	.17
3 Getting Along with Others	3.94	.83	.12	−.18	.54	.42	.31	.14	.14
4 Feelings and Mood	4.31	1.04	.15	−.18	.33	.56	.28	.32	.21
5 Use of Free Time	3.14[a]	1.42	.39	.20	.29	.25	.78	.33	.34
6 Problems	4.22	.99	.38	−.08	.51	.39	.48	.51	.54
7 Attitude toward Self	4.00	1.15	.02	.32	.15	.09	.37	.32	.35

Note: Correlations between ratings on the same scale are italicized.
[a]Means differ significantly, $p \leq 0.05$.

Table 4–10
Correlations between Goal Ratings of Case Managers and Significant Others for Developmentally Disabled Males (N = 38)

Significant Others	X̄	sd	Case Managers						
			1	2	3	4	5	6	7
X̄			3.03	4.08	4.05	4.55	2.87	4.34	4.08
sd			1.28	1.58	.84	.55	1.02	.78	.78
1 Family Interaction	3.08	1.36	.82	.46	.21	.33	.63	.23	.35
2 Occupation	3.63	1.78	.37	.79	.09	.16	.44	.25	.37
3 Getting Along with Others	4.25	.90	.23	.08	.41	.54	.46	.43	.43
4 Feelings and Mood	4.42	.95	.15	.19	.21	.47	.34	.31	.57
5 Use of Free Time	3.11	1.43	.44	.43	.33	.50	.73	.38	.47
6 Problems	4.13	1.04	.16	.06	.08	.38	.25	.31	.48
7 Attitude toward Self	4.08	1.00	.17	.32	.22	.36	.41	.38	.72

Note: Correlations between ratings on the same scale are italicized.

Table 4–11
Correlations between Goal Ratings of Case Managers and Significant Others for Developmentally Disabled Females (N = 36)

Significant Others	X̄	sd	Case Managers						
			1	2	3	4	5	6	7
X̄			3.58	3.92	4.14	4.39	3.25	4.31	4.08
sd			1.13	1.54	.72	.69	1.10	.95	.94
1 Family Interaction	3.86	1.12	.72	.31	.41	.37	.44	.44	.42
2 Occupation	3.86	1.38	.33	.62	.11	.03	.29	.10	.10
3 Getting Along with Others	4.14	.80	.10	.10	.57	.37	.28	.21	.29
4 Feelings and Mood	4.61	.77	.27	.03	.41	.62	.29	.32	.25
5 Use of Free Time	3.56	1.32	.25	.02	.16	.23	.67	.13	.22
6 Problems	4.47	.77	.30	.18	.44	.45	.46	.54	.57
7 Attitude toward Self	4.22	.99	.16	.09	.15	.16	.37	.23	.29

Note: Correlations between ratings on the same scale are italicized.

However, ratings of *Problems* by significant others tend to correlate more highly with ratings of *Attitude Toward Self* by case managers than they do with ratings on the correspondingly named scale. On the basis of these data, one may conclude that the scales show considerable convergent and discriminant validity.

The case managers' ratings of goals tend to be quite close, on the average, to those of the parent or guardian (see tables 4–10 and 4–11). The only significant difference is that for *Occupation* for males, the case managers making the higher average goal rating. For goal ratings as for current-status ratings, there is convincing evidence of convergent validity. Correlations between goal ratings on corresponding scales range from 0.31 to 0.82 for males, with a median of 0.72, and from 0.29 to 0.72 for females, with a median of 0.62. Discriminant validity is, again, somewhat weaker among scales 3, 4, 6, and 7 than among 1, 2, and 5.

Concluding Remarks

It is evident that our data on the use of the PES with the developmentally disabled are somewhat sparser than those that have been collected on the emotionally disturbed population. However, the data that have been obtained indicate that the scales can be used with moderate reliability by raters with two hours of training. Further studies are needed in this area to assess the effect of increased experience on reliability as well as to explore other conditions that may affect ratings, such as the professional background of the rater and the nature of the activities observed. Comparison of ratings made by a parent or guardian with those made by the case managers serving the developmentally disabled client indicates that their perceptions are remarkably similar. These data provided evidence that ratings made by individuals well acquainted with the client display convergent and discriminant validity and thus, inferentially, higher reliability than our earlier data.

PES current-status ratings of mildly to moderately developmentally disabled clients are, for the most part, uncorrelated with age and IQ. One exception to this is the score on *Family Interaction*, which is positively correlated with age for women and with IQ for both men and women. A somewhat greater number of significant correlations were found between goal ratings and age and IQ. In particular, *Occupation* and *Family Interaction* correlated positively with IQ for both sexes, while *Occupation* correlated negatively with age.

Further studies are needed to assess the impact of various programs on clients by means of successive ratings over a period of time.

5 The Heuristic Value of the Progress Evaluation Scales

This chapter focuses on the possible applications of the Progress Evaluation Scales to clinical, programmatic, and administrative and policy questions, as well as to problems of public relations and accountability. The purpose will be to delineate some of the unique issues that can be explored with these scales, not to present an exhaustive list of all questions that can potentially be investigated or situations to which the evaluations can meaningfully be applied. We believe that the system of assessment and evaluation made possible by the PES has some definite advantages over other approaches and should result in at least circumscribed answers to many of the problems that plague therapists and administrators. In particular, it provides the possibility of obtaining continual updated information about one's client population in a manner that is meaningful and pertinent both to the general public and to mental-health professionals. Furthermore, the ease, speed, and low cost with which such information can be obtained should make it possible to collect and maintain its quality over time.

The Clinical Domain

Traditionally research in psychotherapy has focused on questions of outcome and process. These broad domains of inquiry have been further subdivided in terms of impact of therapist variables, patient variables, environmental variables, therapeutic technique variables, and, less frequently, interaction effects. Since relatively little systematic attention has been paid to the role of goal setting in psychotherapy and to the possible uses of outcome data for feedback purposes, we shall examine in some detail possible uses of the PES in these areas. Additionally, we shall provide some examples that illustrate the relevance of the scales to applied clinical-research studies, particularly when these studies involve the combined effect of two or more variables on outcome.

Goal Setting

Meaningful goal setting for community mental-health clients is predicated on the availability of prior, empirically established norms of adjustment for various psychiatric populations. Such norms should reflect acceptable levels of functioning in the community for such populations. Furthermore, norms are also necessary in order to set reasonable goals for program implementation and for assessing the outcome of various intervention approaches. Relying for these purposes on general community norms, which are usually established by assessing the adjustment level of well-functioning groups in the community, is unrealistic for most psychiatric patients and misleading to the public, which is led to believe that mental-health services can produce results that actually occur only rarely. Additionally, use of such general community norms to assess outcome of mental-health services rendered to chronic, low-functioning clients, such as psychotics or serious personality disorders, is unfair, unrealistic, and contributes to "burn-out" among mental-health professionals.

The use of general community norms for outcome criteria is meaningful only for a small segment of the population served by mental-health centers. This population essentially consists of well-adjusted individuals who are temporarily unable to cope with sudden or great stress, such as loss of a job, death of a family member, discovery of an incurable disease in a loved one, and the like. In contrast to these relatively few, well-adjusted individuals who seek help from community mental-health centers, most psychiatric patients seeking help have a history of chronic maladjustment in one or more central roles of their lives (familial, social, vocational). Clinical experience has taught most therapists not to expect psychiatric patients to achieve levels of functioning comparable to those of nonclinical populations in the community, irrespective of the nature and duration of their therapeutic endeavor. Supporting such clinical impressions is a large number of studies conducted over a number of years in the Shiawassee County Community Mental Health Center. These studies indicate, according to ratings of therapists from various professional disciplines and the independent ratings of clients and their significant others, that most community mental-health center clients do not achieve levels of functioning comparable to general community norms upon termination of their treatment. This statement needs to be qualified since we lack follow-up studies to estimate what additional improvement or deterioration occurs over time in these clients. Inasmuch as about a third of all outpatient clients tend to resume treatment in community mental-health centers within three years and about half of those discharged from state institutions are readmitted to psychiatric hospitals, one can assume that for many clients there is substantial deterioration over time. Unfortunately, data for clients who continue to improve after formal psychotherapy ended are generally unavailable.

Using unrealistic community norms as the goals of treatment is detrimental in another way: these goals are bound to lead a cost-conscious public to the conclusion that mental-health services fail to achieve their own reasonable objectives. Since erosion of public support in our society is usually translated into reduced legislative confidence and shrunken fiscal allocations, it is imperative for the field of mental health to establish empirically reasonable norms of adjustment for various psychiatric populations in the community. Such norms should then serve as guidelines for goal setting for different psychiatric populations, as well as become the criteria for realistic assessment of the efficiency and effectiveness of various clinical interventions. Additionally availability of such norms could be used for establishing screening criteria for service, providing an objective basis for making treatment plans, or be used as guides for initiating termination of services. At the present time such determinations are made without established criteria, which makes quality control and meaningful evaluation of services impossible.

In applied clinical research one can use the PES to explore such questions as, What goals can be achieved, over a twelve-month period, in a day-treatment program serving chronic schizophrenics discharged from state institutions? What goals should be set for chronic female alcoholics who attend outpatient group psychotherapy for twelve months?

Of interest to agencies rendering services to children would be to explore such questions as, Is outcome of treatment related to differences in parental perception of their child's current functioning? Is outcome influenced by degree of agreement between the goals set independently by each parent for their child? Is it beneficial to reconcile parental perception of their child's current-functioning level before goals are set?

Another line of inquiry of practical importance concerns the effects of self-fulfilling prophecy on therapeutic outcome. In this regard it would be interesting to explore such questions as, Is outcome for various diagnostic groups related to level of goal setting by therapists, patients, or significant others? Do clients who set high goals for themselves improve more or less compared to clients who set only moderate goals? Does reconciliation of differences in goals set by clients and their therapists affect dropout rate, outcome, or satisfaction with services rendered?

These few examples should suggest the scope and seminal importance of questions that the PES could help explore.

Provision of Feedback

One of the advantages provided by the PES evaluation system is the possibility it affords for giving feedback to interested parties. We shall examine this issue by reviewing four primary areas for provision of feedback. First, we shall examine the question of feedback to clients upon termination of therapy; second, we shall discuss feedback to therapists; third, we shall examine the question of feedback to community referral sources; fourth, we shall see how PES feedback data could be useful for conflict resoution.

Feedback to Clients: A large number of unresolved questions exist in relationship to provision of feedback to clients at termination of psychotherapy. At this juncture it is unclear whether it is beneficial, detrimental, or makes no difference if clients are provided with documented information on what their functioning was when their treatment began; what progress, if any, they have made; which goals were achieved; what a client's current functioning is in relationship to other successfully treated clients with similar conditions; and the like. Will such periodic reviews with clients forestall premature terminations? How will it affect tendencies of "aye-saying" and "nay-saying" in response to follow-up consumer satisfaction questionnaires? Would examining such material be damaging to some clients but beneficial to others?

At the present time, there is no consensus among clinicians whether provision of feedback at termination of therapy is beneficial to all, some, or no clients. However, since decisions related to feedback are continuously being made, we must develop a sound base of knowledge to improve this clinical practice. Although it is unlikely that such investigations could produce any fixed formulas on what to do under various conditions, such an inquiry may, nevertheless, provide useful information to clinicians on how to refine this process of now largely intuitive decision making.

Feedback to Therapists: Feedback to therapists is an area in which very little systematic research has been done. It would be useful to find out, for example, how different therapists in an agency perform with clients who function high and low on various domains measured by the PES (such as occupation, self-esteem, or coping capacity). If, for example, one finds that patients who score low in self-esteem have a particularly high or low dropout rate after an initial interview when seen by a therapist in an agency, it would be beneficial to the field in general to study in depth the nature of the relationships that these therapists establish with such clients. One could explore here such questions as, What are the communication characteristics of therapists who work well with clients with low scores on *Attitude toward Self?* How do interviewers with high dropout rates relate to such clients? Additionally one can ask, Do earlier dropout rates also mean less improvement and less satisfaction with services?

It is reasonable to expect taht some therapists may excel in treating highly dependent clients who score low on *Family Interaction* as well as on self-esteem; these same therapists may find it difficult, however, to treat clients effectively who, although low on self-esteem, are defiantly independent. There probably are therapists who work effectively with both clinical groups. What are their characteristics? Such knowledge can be extremely useful since it may lead to improving the overall efficiency and effectiveness of clinical services. Improvement in this area is especially important in light of the fact that about half of the applicants for community mental-health services drop out within a few sessions, before any of their major goals are achieved.

Feedback to the Community: The attitudes held by agencies and community groups toward providers of mental-health services are of great relevance to community mental-health centers. Periodically community agencies and professionals are surveyed as to whether clients they have referred to the local mental-health center have benefited from services rendered. Unfortunately the respondents to such surveys, with rare exceptions, know very little about the outcome or usefulness of mental-health services. For example, if a client with a long arrest record, who was referred to a community mental-health center by the local district court for counseling, has not been rearrested prior to such a survey, the personnel of the court usually view such a client as a successfully treated referral. Quite frequently, however, the client may have continued to be involved in a life of crime, which the therapist may or may not know about. Without a carefully thought out system for exchange of information, the court can easily misread the rate of success or failure of their referrals. Usually therapists are either required to give detailed reports to courts, which has the effect of forcing their clients to keep them in the dark regarding what is really happening in their lives, or therapists have worked out an agreement with the court whereby they report only attendance records, which in effect keeps the court in the dark regarding the question of impact of mental-health services on the functioning of court-referred clients.

When community agencies lack relevant data on which to base their opinions about the impact of mental-health services, they rarely acknowledge such lack of information. Instead they tend to form opinions on the basis of a variety of personal experiences. One set of important experiences is the quality of informal relationships that the personnel of various agencies maintain with mental-health-center board members, staff, and administrative personnel. These relationships are, in turn, determined by the existence of mutual interests, participation in the same service clubs, churches, and other social or professional organizations. Another important influence on the opinions of community agencies results from service availability in terms of an expeditious referral process, easy access to emergency services during and after work hours, timely preparation of reports for agencies that must meet deadlines of one sort or another (for example, court hearings and disability determinations), and the like.

Central to the question of feedback provision to agencies is the fact that mental-health professionals face a dilemma: they hesitate to provide information on individual clients, since this is bound to turn psychotherapy into a sham; on the other hand, they are hesitant about providing feedback about groups of clients because of the difficulty of demonstrating cause-effect relationships between psychotherapy and certain outcomes. Reports on outcome of mental-health services invariably raise the question of the role of other variables in the therapeutic endeavor, such as extent of emotional support from the family, change in economic conditions, and the like.

Much useful information can be exchanged with referral sources, however, without infringing on client rights to confidentiality and without being caught in the moot question of cause-effect in psychotherapy. For example, quarterly reports can be produced that display data on groups of clients referred by various agencies for mental-health services. These reports can indicate the percentage of clients who have improved, regressed, or remained unchanged since initiation of services. Outcome can be analyzed in terms of overall change in adjustment (sum scores of the seven PES), as well as in more detail, describing change in status on each of the seven dimensions tapped by the PES. While cause-effect relationships between treatment and outcome are hard to prove, and this needs to be made explicit to referral sources, sharing of the best available information has clear advantages. Reports to agencies could contain information on the level of functioning of clients they have referred prior to the beginning of treatment, what their level was when they were reevaluated after six months, and how they functioned at termination of treatment. Such data are especially interesting when examined from the perspective of therapists' perception, the clients' point of view, and that of significant others. Integrating in such analyses various demographic variables, such as age, sex, education, and diagnosis, can enhance understanding by referral sources of what are reasonable expectations to hold for various clients referred to a mental-health agency for service. Community agencies can better appreciate why certain goals are set for various client populations and how to view outcome in light of these goals. Such reports can help clarify to agencies why limited goals (stabilization of functioning) are set for a group of chronic schizophrenic clients, while for other clients the goals set anticipate dramatic improvement (as might be expected in the case of clients with a good history of prior adjustment, who were referred for mental-health consultation because of severe disturbance due to unusually stressful circumstances).

The development of informative, imaginative, and interesting reports for the public is a great challenge to mental-health professionals today; perhaps the very existence of community supported mental-health services is in the balance. A significant advantage of the PES is that they can provide useful data for the preparation of such reports. Finally, PES information, being free of professional jargon and clinical terminology, has the additional advantage of helping to demystify mental illness, a condition still shrouded in the public's mind in ignorance, superstition, and prejudice.

Conflict Management: In the last two decades the number of malpractice suits brought against human-service agencies, and against health professionals in particular, has increased dramatically. The consensus is that this phenomenon is connected to the emergence of a national consumer movement, the general erosion of trust in authority and government, and the disillusionment with the sciences as arbiters of human problems. These social trends are believed to have played an important role in creating a more-assertive, searching, and questioning public. Coexisting with these public attitudes are a broad set of unrealistic expectations on the part of the lay public as to what experts and sciences can and ought to deliver. While excessive expectations in any area are bound to result in disappointments, this is particularly true in the health field, where the impact is always highly personal and frequently stress producing. Many people are still shaken when they find out that various treatment procedures, which they vaguely assumed to be scientifically based, are in fact intuitive; that the best outcome of treatment for different conditions is stabilization at low levels of functioning rather than cure or improvement. Such revelations form a fertile ground for strife, particularly when the relationship between patient and health professional is impersonal and brief, which is more and more the case in our highly mobile society.

In the mental-health field, strife typically occurs when clients, their families, or consumer-advocate groups feel that certain mental-health services were denied or improperly rendered. In outpatient mental-health clinics conflict is likely to occur with coerced referrals (court-ordered evaluations, school-requested assessments, and the like). When treatment is recommended against the client's or the family's wishes, the mental-health professional may become embroiled in a melee of pressure and counterpressures from which it is extremely difficult to extricate oneself with one's professional esteem intact.

It is of paramount importance to the mental-health field to be able to demonstrate with objective evidence how estimates are made regarding the level of psychological functioning of evaluated clients. For example, one should be able to answer such questions as, How was it determined that a client needed or did not need mental-health services? After services have been rendered over a certain period of time, How was it determined whether there has been improvement, no change, or deterioration in the client's functioning? Such seemingly simple and straightforward questions, however, are not easy to answer. It has been our experience that when such queries are posed, they can tax the skill, ingenuity, and credibility of the most knowledgeable and experienced clinician.

We have found that most professionals tend to become defensive or patronizing when their judgment is questioned. They frequently take the position that only other professionals can properly assess the nature of their findings and conclusion, which sometimes is true. Additionally, clinicians tend to resort to jargon-loaded statements to explain their findings and justify their decisions—for example, "The patient, as a result of psychotherapy, successfully decathected his obsessive attachment to his mother and is now capable of libidinizing other, more suitable sex objects." The lay public, in our experience, usually do not respond well to this form of discourse, even when such clinical formulations have dynamic validity and carry significant explanatory power. Since such clinical formulations do not enhance communication with the lay public, a matter of primary concern, perhaps such explanations should be reserved for professional workshops and scientific journals.

On a number of occasions we have found it useful to explain our findings and recommendations by sharing data gathered with the PES. This was especially helpful when we had independent ratings from clients, their significant others, and therapists, filled out at entry and at various points after treatment began. Contrasting such ratings with general community norms and the typical functioning level of various clinical groups carried significant weight in explaining our professional decisions.

Applied Clinical-Evaluation Research

The problems inherent in carrying out applied research in community mental-health settings have been discussed in a number of publications (for example, Cowen, 1978). The use of the PES answers some of the criticisms expressed, such as the need for providing outcome criteria relevant to the goals of community mental-health centers and obtainable from those persons most centrally involved—the client, the therapist and significant others. Although the PES scales offer no panacea for all problems mentioned in the literature, in our judgment some of the problems can be handled better by this system than by other currently existing approaches.

One important area of inquiry concerns formulation of individual treatment plans for clients. Such plans, to be valid, depend on the possession of relevant knowledge as to which interventions work best for which groups of clients. While general accountability-related questions (for example, Is outpatient counseling helpful to emotionally disturbed children?) are important for certain purposes, answers to such questions are not likely to improve the effectiveness of mental-health services. For this purpose a more-complex research strategy is needed, which enables one to contrast the impact of different treatment modalities on groups of clients, matched on specified clinical and demographic characteristics.

To embark upon this kind of inquiry, one must pose such questions as, Is the outcome more satisfactory, over specified time intervals, if married alcoholics are treated in a couples' group psychotherapy as compared to conjoint marital therapy? Is the outcome more satisfactory when female therapists, rather than equally competent male therapists, treat emotionally disturbed girls of a particular age group and diagnostic category? The answers to such questions can yield relevant information for improving the efficiency and effectiveness of clinical services.

There are many such unanswered questions that plague the mental-health field. Their exploration in one agency may yield only locally optimal answers, but the combined answers from many centers could result in the satisfactory resolution of such issues or reveal what other conditions must be taken into account.

The Programmatic Domain

For an assessment to be useful in the area of program evaluation, it is first necessary to delineate the kind and level of questions that are to be subsumed under this domain. We propose that issues requiring decision making at the level of program or agency director be classified under this category. These issues encompass questions of selection of methodology for desired program outcome, cost-benefit analysis, quality control, assignment of staff, utilization of results for feedback purposes, and the like.

At this level one could explore such questions as, Which intervention methods (for example, insight-oriented group psychotherapy or individual behavior therapy) in a particular program area (perhaps aftercare or substance abuse) produce the most satisfactory results, at lowest cost, over certain time intervals? Which clinical populations respond best to certain therapeutic interventions—for example, desensitization, biofeedback, gestalt psychotherapy? What additional resources, available in most communities, such as volunteers, can augment program implementation and lead to better outcome? Does frequency of service rendered (for example, one versus two therapy sessions per week) to certain client groups (for example, inadequate personalities) make a differential impact on their level of adjustment over a specified time interval? Does the allocation of additional resources improve program impact or provide the same outcome at increased cost? At what cost is progress achieved from one level of functioning, on a particular dimension of the PES, to the next level? While the exploration of such questions can potentially improve program performance, it will no doubt require extensive and consistent replication of certain results before trust could be placed in a particular intervention strategy.

Another important use of PES data in the programmatic domain is that they may alert agency directors to changing characteristics in the population being served. Such changes, such as a significant increase in number of clients requiring services regarding occupational difficulties, may require outreach programs to employers, training of therapists in new service modalities, development of special seminars for the staff of other human-service agencies in the community, and the like. Finally, we have found that the use of the PES for consultation purposes can help reconcile differences in perception among the staff of various agencies working with the same clients, thus leading to a more-consistent intervention strategy.

The Administrative and Policy Domain

The major influence on administrative and policy regulations of local mental-health agencies comes from rules and regulations promulgated by states and the federal government; these areas may include selection of programs for funding, data to be collected, and services to be cut when funding is reduced. Another influence on agency operations is exerted by guidelines issued by various accreditation bodies, such as the Joint Commission on Accreditation of Hospitals and third-pary payers. A more subtle but nevertheless important influence is exerted by the ethnic, cultural, religious, and socioeconomic composition of the population being served, expressed through the views, attitudes, and voting power of community-appointed board members, as well as through the influence of the formal (for example, courts, police, public health) and informal (for example, physicians, lawyers, ministers) community systems, the local news media, influential citizens, and the like.

Contrary to generally held beliefs, the influence of mental-health professionals on fundamental policies affecting mental-health services has been greatly overrated. For example, it is evident that a remarkable shift has taken place in the service priorities of community mental-health

centers. These include a deemphasis on early screening, limited consultation with schools, lack of outreach to children of severely mentally ill
adults, and hardly any consultation with industry regarding employees'
mental-health needs. Most mental-health centers are no longer pursuing
the original goals and objectives of community mental-health services.
Instead, most community mental-health centers have turned into agencies
designed to provide support services to low-functioning, deinstutionalized
clients through a variety of day programs, medication clinics, case-man-
agement services, residential programs, socialization groups, and the
like. A recent survey of community mental-health centers in Michigan,
for example, revealed that little was being done now in the areas of
consultation, screening, or prevention. The findings indicate that 88 percent of the community mental-health centers in Michigan are doing no
outreach to children of severely mentally ill adults; 83 percent reported
no systematic screening of county jail inmates for presence of mental
illness; only about 1 percent of the mental-health budget was earmarked
for prevention services. The priorities imposed by most states on community mental-health centers are largely dictated by short-range economic
considerations. Since we do not know yet enough about the ultimate value
of prevention, consultation, and outreach, these services are likely to
disappear altogether unless convincing studies can be presented to clarify
the long-range effects of such programs. Unfortunately, very few high-
quality, long-range studies in these areas are being conducted at the
present time. The possible application of the different versions of the
PES to children, adolescents, and adults, using the same seven dimensions
of adjustment, can be especially useful in longitudinal studies.

There is a general consensus that mental-health professionals have
had limited influence on the fundamental policies affecting their field.
Their opinions are suspect as self-serving, and this has too often proven
to be the case; their lack of relevant, objective data with which to make
a case has been evident to all. Perhaps the major contribution that mental-
health professionals can make for the adoption of sound policies and
priorities in the mental-health field is through collection and presentation
of data relevant to policies under consideration. Until such data are available, it is hard to see how present trends can be influenced, much less
reversed.

Considering the public need to make the best possible use of its
resources, it is imperative that a meaningful data base be developed for
mental-health services. At this juncture we still lack the information
necessary to answer such questions as, Is there evidence that the clients
one proposes to serve derive long-range benefit from the kind of program
for which funds are requested? Does a proposed philosophy of service
enhance family cohesiveness, independence, and self-respect? Is there

a long-term fiscal or other community advantage in supporting a proposed intervention strategy?

While we would not be so presumptive as to suggest that the Progress Evaluation Scales can yield the full answer to such all-encompassing questions, we propose nevertheless that they can generate relevant information, which can be weighed with other considerations in the decision-making process in determining policy at various levels of responsibility.

Appendix A
Administration and
Scoring Procedures

Instructions for Initial-Status Rating and Goal Setting

General Instructions

Raters should be aware of the definitions of the seven PES scales and the special instructions for rating each scale.

Raters should familiarize themselves with the five items that make up each of the seven scales of the PES forms before they interview clients. (Such familiarity is a precondition for eliciting the required information during the diagnostic interview for reliable use of the scales.)

Before undertaking the routine use of the PES, it is desirable to interview a client in the presence of another rater or sit in on an interview conducted by another rater. (Comparing independently made ratings and discussing differences in marked items was found to alert interviewers to idiosyncrasies in their interpretation of PES items.)

Rating of clients on the PES should be made on the basis of observed behavior and reported experience and not on the basis of any particular theory. For example, if an obese patient indicates in the interview that he likes himself as a person and reports feeling positively about himself most of the time, he is to be rated highly on the *Attitude toward Self* scale, even though psychoanalytic theory may postulate that he has low self-esteem because obese patients allegedly make themselves unattractive by putting on excess weight; ipso facto, they must have low self-esteem, which is unconsciously driving them to overeat and look unattractive. On the other hand, when a client verbally denies problems for which reliable evidence exists, such as loss of jobs due to alcoholism, the interviewer makes the ratings on the basis of the best available information.

Instructions for Rating Current Functioning

The initial rating of current functioning and goals is completed at the end of the diagnostic interview. To complete the PES properly, interviewers must first familiarize themselves with their client's background, life-style, and functioning on the dimensions tapped by the scales. For the purpose of rating *Current Functioning* (form 1 of the PES), initial status is defined as "behavior and experience that describes best how the client functioned within the two weeks preceding the evaluation interview."

In making a rating on a particular scale, the item chosen should reflect that client's typical level of functioning on the dimension tapped by that scale. For example, a client who is regularly able to groom and dress properly but sometimes needs help, perhaps in tying shoes is rated above the level of "Requires help with basic needs" (level 1). Similarly, if an individual cannot manage some aspect of a basic need, though overall she functions at a satisfactory level on that dimension—perhaps she can dress well but is unable to tie her shoes—she should be rated at her general level of functioning and not at the level where some limited aspect of a general dimension is malfunctioning. In other words, the person who by and large can dress alone, feed herself, and attend to other personal necessities is rated above the level of needing help with basic needs.

Another aspect the interviewer needs to keep in mind when assessing a client's current level of functioning is the community norms for that age group. For example, a disturbed adult male client who does not hold a job and has to reside in a group home because he is unable to manage his own affairs—that is, he is unable to plan independently his daily activities and unable to care independently for a home or apartment—will be rated at a low level on the *Occupation* scale, even if he cooperates making his bed daily in the group home, helps washing dishes after dinner, helps straighten the house, and so forth. An essential consideration to keep in mind is the fact that this client is unable to maintain an independent living arrangement due to personal, social, and/or occupational difficulties (in contrast to clients who can maintain an independent living arrangement while on welfare, SSI, and similar programs, in which case they are usually rated at higher levels).

To take another example, if a child or adolescent fails half of all her school subjects due to severe emotional disturbance and is subsequently placed in a special class for emotionally impaired, her assessment on the dimension of school functioning *(Occupation)* should be made against the norms of the child's age group (that is, "Cannot pass 50 percent of regular school subjects for his or her age level"), and not on the basis of the child's standing in the special class setting. A teacher's report in a day-treatment program that a 14-year-old child "makes good progress with first-grade reading" is academically and clinically important and should be recorded in the child's chart; it will, nevertheless, place the child at a low level of academic functioning on the PES, which shows that child's functioning in comparison to community norms for that age group, not in relation to the special group the child has been placed in.

Instructions for Setting Goals

After initial-status ratings are made on the seven PES scales, goals are set on a separate sheet (form 2). Form 1 and form 2 are identical except for the instructions. Form 2 instructs that goals be selected in each column for a predetermined number of months. The time frame chosen to achieve certain goals can be varied across populations served, program methodologies, therapeutic techniques, and the like.

In setting goals, interviewers need to weigh: client characteristics (for example, motivation for change, chronicity of psychopathology), environmental constraints (for example, economic conditions, social opportunities), and therapy variables (for example, effectiveness of therapeutic techniques for a particular psychopathology, such as behavior therapy's known effectiveness for enuresis and the lack of any known effective interventions for pedophilia).

Due to the limited knowledge about the differential effectiveness of various therapeutic techniques and due to the fact that the prevailing termination rates within the first ten sessions reach 70 percent in most mental-health centers, it is recommended that the following periods be used for goal setting when routine evaluation is made for clients seeking mental-health services:

1. For outpatient clients who do not have a chronic history of low level of functioning, goals should be initially set for a three-month period; clients who are still in active treatment after three months are to be reevaluated and new goals set for the next six months; similarly, six-month goals are to be set at each review period thereafter, for as long as these clients receive outpatient therapeutic services.

2. For clients who are being enrolled in rehabilitation services, such as, sheltered workshop, sheltered employment, and other similar programs, which are designed to improve the adjustment of chronically low-functioning clients, initial and subsequent goals are to be set for six-month periods, for as long as clients attend these programs.

3. For clients who are being enrolled in maintenance programs (day activity services, walk-in medication review clinics, and so forth), for whom minimal progress is anticipated, initial and subsequent goals are to be set for twelve months, for as long as clients are enrolled in these programs.

Instructions for Administering the PES to Adults, Adolescents, Children, and the Developmentally Disabled

Following are the procedures for administering the PES to clients.

Adults: First, it is ascertained that a client can read at a level of comprehending a newspaper article; then he or she is given form 1 and form 2 of the PES scales (*Current Functioning* and *Goals*), stapled one to the other. The therapist then freely paraphrases the instructions printed on the upper-left-hand corner of the forms. The clients are told that they are to read all the items in the first column of the evaluation form and then select the one item in that column that best describes their behavior during the past two weeks, by circling that item. After they complete the first column, they are to proceed to the other six columns on the page, in a similar fashion. If clients have no questions at this point, they are instructed that upon completion of the first page (form 1), they are to turn to the second page (form 2), but that this time the items they select should represent realistic goals for their therapy for the number of months indicated on the form.

If after reading a column, a patient complains that none of the items in that column describes him or her well, the interviewer should acknowledge that sometimes none of the items fits an individual well but that the interviewer would appreciate it if the client reviewed the items further and chose the one that describes him or her the best. When this happens, it is advisable to encourage clients to write down their reservations in the "Comments" section, on the bottom of the PES form. If the client does not respond to this additional effort at persuasion, further urging is usually not desirable from a clinical standpoint, and the form is to be treated as "Incomplete" (the procedures for handling incomplete forms are described below).

If the adult client did not learn to read or is mentally or emotionally disturbed to the point of being unable to follow the instructions for filling out the PES forms, then a family member or a guardian who is familiar with the client's daily behavior and problems should be asked to do the ratings for the client.

Children and Adolescents: If the client is an adolescent (age 13 through 17), it is first ascertained that he or she can read at a level of comprehending a newspaper article; then the client and the client's significant others (mother and father, if both are available) are given Adolescent Forms of *Current Functioning* and *Goals* to fill out independently. If the client is a child (age 6 through 12), only significant others are asked to fill out the Children's Forms of the PES.

If the significant others are mentally disturbed to the point of being unable to fill out the forms, another family member or a guardian who is familiar with the child's or adolescent's problems and daily behavior should be asked to do the ratings.

When significant others fill out the PES, the therapist marks on the form the relationship of that significant other to the client (mother, father, sister, uncle, and so on).

Developmentally Disabled: Developmentally disabled are defined as clients coming under the Developmentally Disabled Act Amendments of 1978, PL95-602. The studies reported on developmentally disabled in this book, however, covered only mentally retarded clients. When these clients are enrolled in programs, their significant others or guardians are given Developmentally Disabled Forms of *Current Functioning* and *Goals* to fill out. If the significant other or guardian is mentally disturbed to the point of being unable to follow the instructions for filling out the form, another family member or person familiar with the client's life-style and problems is asked to do the ratings on the client.

Instructions for Handling Incomplete Ratings

If a patient or a significant other is not completing the PES scales, the therapist circles the reason on the incompleted forms in accordance with the following code, which is printed on the upper-right-hand corner of the PES form:

CR—cannot read.

TD—too disturbed (for example, hallucinates).

DX—seen for diagnostic purposes only (for example, presentencing evaluation for court).

UA—unavailable (usually occurs at reevaluation or termination).

OT—other reasons (for example, refuses).

Example: Client: CR (TD) DX UA OT
         Significant: Other CR TD DX (UA) OT

Instructions for Reevaluation Procedures

General Instructions

All clients are reevaluated by their assigned therapists or case managers if they are still receiving service at the time their reevaluation is due. The reevaluation date is determined by the number of months for which goals are set. All clinicians complete reevaluation forms on the basis of their overall knowledge of their clients' functioning, as reflected in the progress notes maintained by the clinical staff, mail and phone communications with clients' families, and the like. Clients may or may not be asked to fill out reevaluation forms, depending upon the nature of the evaluation program, client availability, and the like.

If a client terminates services prior to his or her reevaluation date, a closing evaluation is completed by clinicians and a PES form is mailed to clients for completion.

In addition to having therapists and case managers reevaluate all of their clients, a representative sample can be selected from each population of clients served to be reevaluated independently by a second clinician. This second evaluation is performed on the basis of a face-to-face interview with clients and/or their significant others.

If a client is transferred from one program to another (for example, from outpatient to sheltered workshop), a closing evaluation is completed for the program from which the client exits, and an initial evaluation is made by the new program staff.

A client who is enrolled in two programs or more is reevaluated in each program, based on the time frame set to achieve certain goals in that program area.

Instructions for Reevaluating Outpatient,
Rehabilitation, and Maintenance Clients

All outpatient clients are reevaluated by their therapists if they are still receiving outpatient services three months after the diagnostic interview. At that point, new six-month goals are set. For clients not in treatment any longer during the reevluation period (defined as three months of no contact with outpatient services), a closing evaluation is completed. These reevaluations and closing evaluations by primary therapists and case managers are not necessarily based on face-to-face interviews with their clients. Therapists make these ratings on the basis of their general knowledge of their clients' status as is reflected in their progress notes, as well as from whatever additional information they possess from telephone or mail contact, from contacts with the clients' families, and the like.

All clients still being served in rehabilitation programs six months after their initial enrollment are reevaluated by their supervisor or case manager; at that point, new six-month goals are set. If clients are not being served any longer (defined as six months of no contact with the program), closing evaluations are completed.

All clients still being served in maintenance programs twelve months after their initial enrollment are reevaluated by their therapists or case managers; at that point, new twelve-month goals are set. If clients are not being served any longer (defined as twelve months of no contact with the program), a closing evaluation is completed.

Evaluation at Termination of Services

The records of outpatient clients who have had no face-to-face contact with the agency staff over a three-month period are routinely closed. For clients enrolled in rehabilitation programs, a six-month period is used; for clients in maintenance programs, a twelve-month period is allowed. However, if a client moves out of the catchment area or dies, the record is closed forthwith. Therapists rate the clients' functioning on the PES at time of closing based on their progress notes, telephone conversations with clients, and whatever other contact they may have had with their clients' families over the phone, in person, or by mail.

All clients whose cases are being closed are mailed a consumer satisfaction questionnaire and form 1 of the PES *(Current Functioning)*. A cover letter explains the purpose of mailing these forms and requests the clients to complete the materials and return them in a stamped, self-addressed envelope which is provided. Return rate has been about 30 percent, which is similar to that reported in other consumer satisfaction questionnaire studies.

Reevaluations of Representative Samples

Choice of Representative Samples

Since it is unlikely that sufficient resources will ever be available to public or private agencies for the purpose of tracking down and reevaluating every recipient of mental-health services, the most-reasonable alternative for maintaining quality control requires the selection and reevaluation of representative samples of clients. Representative samples can be formed based on demographic variables such as age (for example, children, adolescents, adults), program areas (for example, aftercare, substance-abuse), diagnosis (for example, neurosis, psychosis), treatment modality (for example, behavior therapy, cognitive therapy), and the like.

The number and size of samples an agency selects for follow-up will usually depend upon the purpose of the study, the nature of the population served by that agency, the resources available to the agency, and general statistical considerations.

General Instructions for Reevaluation of Representative Samples

When reevaluations are due, clients from the special samples are contacted by their assigned clinician (other than the primary therapist). That staff person introduces himself or herself to the client and explains the purpose of the call, which is to set up an appointment at a mutually convenient time for reevaluation purposes. If a client has no telephone, a letter is mailed in which the client is asked to call the agency clinician for an appointment regarding reevaluation. Clients are informed that no fee will be charged for that session. If a client is not reached within a month or refuses to participate, this is recorded (for analysis purposes), and a different client is selected for the sample, following the established criteria (that is, a new client who belongs to the sampled population is drawn from the registry book by choosing the person who falls above the client who dropped out; if that person cannot be reached or if he or she refuses to participate, the client falling below the person who dropped out is contacted; this process is continued until the person is replaced). In a preliminary study, 92 percent of clients reached by our nurse to set an appointment for reevaluation agreed to participate.

Clients in Treatment

If a client from the special sample is still in treatment at the time of the face-to-face reevaluation, a rating of *Current Functioning* is made and new six- or twelve-month goals are set, both by client and the assigned clinician. (If the client is not in treatment any longer, a closing rating is made using only the *Current Functioning* form.) For clients who were unable to complete the PES during the diagnostic interview because they could not read, refused to cooperate, or some other reason, the same significant other, if possible, should be asked to complete the reevaluation forms; if that client can complete the scales now, he or she is encouraged to do so.

Termination of Services

Those patients selected to represent the populations served by the agency, who have had no face-to-face contact with the mental-health center staff for three, six, or twelve months (for outpatient, rehabilitation, and maintenance clients), have their records closed. Clients in the special samples, however, are invited for an interview with an assigned agency clinician (other than their primary therapist). When contacted, they are given the option of having the interview conducted at the agency or in their own home. (The latter option has been chosen very infrequently by outpatients; whether rehabilitation or maintenance clients have different preferences has not been ascertained as yet.)

Since for many clients in the special sample, the closing evaluation is also the first reevaluation (this is usually the case for all clients treated for fewer than three months), the introduction of the assigned clinician and the purpose of the closing evaluation need to be done with special care, with ample opportunity provided to clients to ask questions about reasons for the evaluation, possible expense, time required, and so forth.

No fee should be charged the client for the closing evaluation interview initiated by the agency. At the end of the interview the client and the clinician each complete only form 1 of the PES *(Current Functioning)*; the client is also given on that occasion the consumer satisfaction questionnaire to fill out.

Follow-up Evaluation

The samples selected to represent the various populations served by the agency are contacted one year after the closing evaluation was performed, for an additional reevaluation. Again, a clinician other than the primary therapist interviews the client either on the agency premises or in the client's home; a fee is not charged for this session either. The interviewer and the client complete form 1 of the PES scale *(Current Functioning)*. With this, the cycle of initial evaluation, reevaluation(s), closing evaluation, and follow-up evaluation is completed for the representative samples.

Scoring Procedures

For purposes of statistical analysis, the five items in each column of the PES are assigned the numerical value of 1 to 5; 1 is keyed to the most pathological level of functioning (top item) and 5 to the healthiest level of functioning (bottom item in the column).

Clinical Guidelines for Rating the PES

The next section presents a guide for rating adults, adolescents, children, and the developmentally disabled. For each of the five levels of the seven PES scales, clinical examples are given to illustrate the basis for the rating decisions. Brief definitions for each of the seven dimensions of the PES are followed by special instructions for rating that scale.

Adults

Family Interaction: This scale taps the dimension of dependence-independence-interdependence; it is assessing the client's level of functioning in the home environment, irrespective of whether the home is his or her family home, a group home, a foster home, or another kind of living arrangement.

Levels	Scale Items	Clinical Examples
Level 1	Often must have help with basic needs (for example, feeding, dressing, toilet).	"Doesn't dress himself in the morning . . . claims Christ instructed him to stay in bed all day."
Level 2	Takes care of own basic needs but must have help with everyday plans and activities.	"I just don't seem to be doing anything . . . I rock and smoke and watch TV all day."
Level 3	Makes own plans but without considering the needs of other family members.	"I work hard all week . . . I am entitled to get drunk on Saturday . . . besides, taking care of the kids is *her* job."
Level 4	Tries to consider everyone's needs but somehow decisions and actions do not work well for everybody in the family.	"I do my best . . . but things don't work out the way I mean them."
Level 5	Usually plans and acts so that own needs as well as needs of others in the family are considered.	"No real problems . . . we get along fine."

Occupation (School-Job-Homemaking): This scale taps a person's level of functioning in his or her primary occupational role. When a person is temporarily laid off, or out of school due to vacation, or otherwise not performing the role temporarily, the rating should reflect that person's regular functioning and not the temporary condition he or she is in during the evaluation period (as long as the interviewer is convinced that these circumstances are temporary and not due to client's behavior or attitude).

Levels	Scale Items	Clinical Examples
Level 1	Does not hold job, or care for home, or go to school.	"I am too nervous to go back to work."
Level 2	Seldom holds job, or attends classes, or cares for home.	"Every time I get a job, it never seems to work out."

Level 3	Sometimes holds job, or attends some classes, or does limited housework.	"Have a backache . . . I can't work now in construction, but I pick up odd jobs."
Level 4	Holds regular job, or classes, or does housework (or some combination of these), but with difficulty.	"I hate to get up in the morning because I know I have to go to work and face all those responsibilities."
Level 5	Holds regular job, or attends classes, or does housework (or some combination of these) with little or no difficulty.	"I like my job, am successful, and enjoy the people I work with."

Getting Along with Others: This scale is designed to tap the dimension of socialization. It assesses the quality of relationships established with people outside one's family circle. (Note that this scale does not attempt to differentiate the hostile person from the recluse; both are considered equally unsocialized.)

Levels	*Scale Items*	*Clinical Examples*
Level 1	Always fighting or destructive; or always alone.	"I was hurt by people . . . now I stay away . . . have no friends."
Level 2	Seldom able to get along with others without quarreling or being destructive; or is often alone.	"I'd just as soon not go anywhere . . . 'cause I find it uncomfortable talking to people."
Level 3	Sometimes quarreling, but seldom destructive; difficulties in making friends.	"I visit acquaintances or relatives but I feel out of place . . . it's hard for me to make friends."
Level 4	Gets along with others most of the time; has occasional close friends.	"I have a friend, but I wish I had more people I would be close to."

| Level 5 | Gets along with others most of the time; has regular close friends. | "I have several good friends . . . do things together . . . any one of them would be very helpful in an emergency." |

Feelings and Mood: This scale taps the level of affective modulation as indicated by the degree to which feelings are flexibly expressed and adaptively integrated into overall personality functioning. Careful evaluation is needed of the client's emotional status both during the diagnostic interview and from the client's reports about his or her feelings in a variety of personal and social situations.

Levels	*Scale Items*	*Clinical Examples*
Level 1	Almost always feels nervous, or depressed, or angry and bitter, or no emotions at all.	"I feel empty and numb most of the time . . . I am too nervous."
Level 2	Often feels nervous, or depressed or angry and bitter, or hardly shows any emotion for weeks at a time.	"I feel like nobody gives a damn about me anymore . . . I've been depressed on and off for almost a month now."
Level 3	Frequently in a good mood but occasionally feels nervous, or depressed, or angry for days at a time.	"Used to feel fine most of the time . . . but for the last few days I feel like I am going to explode."
Level 4	Usually in a good mood, but occasionally feels nervous or unhappy, or angry all day.	"Only once in awhile I have down days . . . especially when I don't handle the kids very well.
Level 5	In a good mood most of the time, and usually able to be as happy, or sad, or angry as the situation calls for.	"I've really been feeling good lately . . . no problem with expressing my real feelings."

Use of Free Time: This scale is designed to measure the degree to which

sublimatory processes have satisfactorily evolved by indicating how free
or constricted a person is in using inner and outer resources for play and
enjoyment. In rating the client on this scale, the interviewer should bear
in mind that hobbies and recreational activities may satisfactorily be
engaged in alone or with other people.

Levels	*Scale Items*	*Clinical Examples*
Level 1	Almost no recreational activities or hobbies.	"Nothing seems to interest me anymore . . . when I get home from work, I eat and go to bed."
Level 2	Only occasional recreational activities, or repeats the same activity over and over again.	"I have a couple of TV programs I watch . . . once in a while I play golf in the summer."
Level 3	Participates in some recreational activities or hobbies.	"I like to bowl once or twice a month . . . I plan to join a ceramics class soon."
Level 4	Often participates in recreational activities and hobbies.	"I am taking tennis lessons and I bowl regularly with my wife and two other couples."
Level 5	Participates in, as well as creates, variety of own recreational activities and hobbies for self and others.	"I enjoy reading; like to work with wood as a hobby . . . I like to take the family to shows and picnics."

Problems: This scale was designed to tap the coping capacity the person
can bring to bear on daily problems. At the lowest level of functioning
the person is unable to handle even mild problems; hence, he or she
experiences severe difficulties most of the time. At the highest level of
functioning, the individual is able to handle well even severe problems;
therefore, he or she is described as having only occasionally mild problems. ("Severe" refers to problems that are incapacitating in important
areas, such as homemaking, work, sex, communication, or parenting;
"moderate" refers to problems that are impairing one's efficiency and/
or effectiveness but are not totally incapacitating; "mild" refers to problems that are "annoying or inconveniencing" but do not incapacitate or
interfere with a person's functioning in important areas in their lives.)

Levels	Scale Items	Clinical Examples
Level 1	Severe problems most of the time.	"I am drunk most of the time . . . can't hold a job."
Level 2	Severe problems some of the time or moderate problems continuously.	"I get very tense sometimes and I have to leave work for the day . . . but my boss understands and allows me to make up the time."
Level 3	Moderate problems most of the time, or mild problems almost continuously.	"Frequently I can't concentrate on my work, so I take a walk; if it doesn't help, a couple of aspirins do it for me."
Level 4	Occasional moderate problems.	"Sometimes I get unreasonable, bitchy, irritable, dissatisfied with everything . . . but a hug and a reassuring word help a lot to calm me down."
Level 5	Occasional mild problems.	"Sometimes things don't work out too well, but after I sleep on my problems I usually come up with a solution."

Attitude toward Self: This scale is designed to tap the dimension of self-esteem in terms of the balance of negative and positive attitudes expressed about the self. Clients are rated on the basis of how they report feeling about themselves and not on the basis of inferential deductions derived from theory. For example, if an overweight female client likes herself and has a positive attitude, she is to be rated highly on the *Attitude toward Self* scale, even though psychoanalytic theory might suggest that her obesity is indicative of a low self-esteem. (Since overweight makes her appear unattractive, which leads to social rejection, the theory might postulate that she feels low self-esteem, which is unconsciously driving her to overeat and be rejected.)

Levels	Scale Items	Clinical Examples
Level 1	Negative attitude toward self most of the time.	"I am no good . . . I don't see how anybody could love me."

Level 2	Negative attitude toward self much of the time.	"Much of the time I feel like I am going to fail before I start."
Level 3	Almost equal in positive and negative attitude toward self.	"I feel good about myself at work . . . but I feel crummy when I am at a party or with friends . . . I have nothing to say."
Level 4	Positive attitude toward self much of the time.	"Generally, I feel good about myself . . . though sometimes I wonder."
Level 5	Positive attitude toward self most of the time.	"Most of the time I feel good. I really like myself now."

Adolescents

Family Interaction: This scale taps the dimension of dependence-independence-interdependence; it is assessing the adolescent's level of functioning in his or her home environment, irrespective of whether the home is a family home, a foster home, or another kind of living arrangement.

Levels	*Scale Items*	*Clinical Examples*
Level 1	Often must have help with basic needs (for example, feeding, dressing, toilet).	"I have to help him get dressed for school each morning."
Level 2	Takes care of own basic needs but must have help with everyday plans and activities.	"If I didn't plan everything, she would just sit around all day."
Level 3	Makes own plans but without considering the needs of other family members.	"Even though I ask, plead, threaten . . . he never tells me where he is going to be . . . he is most inconsiderate."
Level 4	Tries to consider everyone's needs but somehow decisions and actions do not work well for everybody in the family.	"She wants to cooperate, but no matter how hard she tries, she just can't seem to get along with her father."

| Level 5 | Usually plans and acts so that own needs as well as needs of others in the family are considered. | "Responsible boy . . . makes a promise and sticks with it." |

Occupation (School-Job-Homemaking): This scale assesses an adolescent's primary occupational role in school, job, or home in comparison to normative functioning for his or her age level. When an adolescent is temporarily out of school, for example, due to vacation, sickness, or other reason, the rating should reflect that adolescent's regular functioning and not the temporary condition he or she is in during the evaluation period (as long as the interviewer is convinced that these circumstances are temporary and not due to the adolescent's behavior or attitude).

Levels	*Scale Items*	*Clinical Examples*
Level 1	Expelled from school, or dropped out of school and holds no job.	"Just hangs around all day . . . ain't interested in anything . . . I am afraid she'll turn into a bum!"
Level 2	Often skips school, or fails most subjects, or seldom holds job.	"I never know if he is going to get to school in the morning or not . . . he just can't catch on."
Level 3	Some school skipping, but passes most subjects, or sometimes holds job.	"She passes most subjects, but could do better . . . school isn't her main interest."
Level 4	Regular school attendance and passes all subjects, or holds regular job (or some combination of these), but with difficulty.	"We had to get a tutor for math, but other than that he is doing OK."
Level 5	Regular school attendance and passes all subjects, or holds regular job (or some combination of these), with little or no difficulty.	"She's doing real well in school . . . tries her best and is well liked."

Getting Along with Others: This scale is designed to tap the dimension of socialization. It assesses the quality of relationships established with peers outside one's family circle. (Note that this scale does not attempt to differentiate the hostile adolescent from the recluse; both are considered equally unsocialized.)

Levels	Scale Items	Clinical Examples
Level 1	Always fighting or destructive; or always alone.	"He has no friends . . . spends all his time in his room . . . can't be with anyone without picking a fight."
Level 2	Seldom able to get along with others without quarreling or being destructive; or is often alone.	"She wants friends . . . but fights and argues a lot so I gather most kids don't want anything to do with her."
Level 3	Sometimes quarreling, but seldom destructive; difficulties in making friends.	"He doesn't make friends easily . . . is shy and stays away from others when he really wants to be with them."
Level 4	Gets along with others most of the time; has occasional close friends.	"She gets along but doesn't get very close . . . now she has one girl she is with constantly, but no one else."
Level 5	Gets along with others most of the time; has regular close friends.	"He is always bringing friends over . . . he has good friends."

Feelings and Mood: This scale taps the level of affective modulation as indicated by the degree to which feelings are flexibly expressed and adaptively integrated into overall personality functioning. Careful observation is needed of the adolescent's emotional status during the diagnostic interview, as well as evaluation of the significant others' reports about the adolescent's feelings in a variety of personal and social situations.

Levels	Scale Items	Clinical Examples
Level 1	Almost always feels nervous, or depressed, or angry and bitter, or no emotions at all.	"There is never any expression on his face to let me know how he feels."

Level 2	Often feels nervous, or depressed, or angry and bitter, or hardly shows any emotion for weeks at a time.	"I've seen her fall apart when she wasn't invited to a party . . . she stays depressed for weeks when she feels rejected."
Level 3	Frequently in a good mood but occasionally feels nervous, or depressed, or angry for days at a time.	"He can go on an emotional bender for days."
Level 4	Usually in a good mood, but occasionally feels nervous, or unhappy, or angry all day.	"She has her bad days . . . doesn't everyone?"
Level 5	In a good mood most of the time, and usually able to be as happy, or sad or angry as the situation calls for.	"Seems pretty comfortable with his emotions . . . is happy most of the time."

Use of Free Time: This scale is designed to measure the degree to which sublimatory processes have satisfactorily evolved by indicating how free or constricted an adolescent is in his use of inner and outer resources for play and enjoyment. In rating the client on this scale, the interviewer should bear in mind that hobbies and recreational activities may satisfactorily be engaged in alone or with other people.

Levels	*Scale Items*	*Clinical Examples*
Level 1	Almost no recreational activities or hobbies.	"Appears to be bored most of the time . . . nothing interests her . . . just sits around."
Level 2	Only occasional recreational activities, or repeats the same activity over and over again.	"All she does day after day is ride her bike and watch TV at night."
Level 3	Participates in some recreational activities or hobbies.	"He sometimes plays ball if the neighbor kids invite him."

| Level 4 | Often participates in recreational activities and hobbies. | "Has been on the swim team each year since eighth grade . . . likes to go hiking with friends." |
| Level 5 | Participates in, as well as creates, variety of own recreational activities and hobbies. | "Likes sports, reading . . . sometimes even organizes the neighborhood football game . . . always has something to do; I never see him bored." |

Problems: This scale was designed to tap the coping capacity the adolescent can bring to bear on daily problems. At the lowest level of functioning, the adolescent is unable to handle even mild problems; hence, he or she experiences severe difficulties most of the time. At the highest level of functioning, the adolescent is able to handle well even severe problems; therefore, he or she is described as having only occasionally mild problems. ("Severe" refers to problems that are incapacitating in important areas, such as school, work, play, or communication; "moderate" refers to problems that are impairing one's efficiency and/or effectiveness but are not totally incapacitating; "mild" refers to problems that are annoying or inconveniencing but do not incapacitate or interfere with his or her functioning in important areas.)

Levels	*Scale Items*	*Clinical Examples*
Level 1	Severe problems most of the time.	"She just goes from one crisis to another . . . doesn't talk to her dad . . . . . . skips school . . . you name it."
Level 2	Severe problems some of the time or moderate problems continuously.	"Feels deeply hurt . . . sometimes for a good reason but not always."
Level 3	Moderate problems most of the time, or mild problems almost continuously.	"Things seem to be on her mind . . . wants to try new things but is scared . . . lacks confidence."
Level 4	Occasional moderate problems.	"School is occasionally a problem, but nothing very serious."
Level 5	Occasional mild problems.	"No real problems . . . just the usual squabble about boyfriends."

Attitude toward Self: This scale is designed to tap the dimension of self-esteem in terms of the balance of negative and positive attitudes expressed about the self. Adolescents are rated on the basis of observations in the diagnostic interview as well as on the basis of reports from self and significant others about how they feel in a variety of situations (with friends, academically, in sports, and so forth) and not on the basis of inferential deductions derived from theory. For example, if a "hyperactive" adolescent boy likes himself and has a positive attitude, he is to be rated highly on the *Attitude toward Self* scale, even though psychoanalytic theory might suggest that his restlessness is indicative of low self-esteem. (Since restlessness in school leads to personal and social difficulties, the theory might postulate that the adolescent has low self-esteem, which is unconsciously driving him to misbehave and be punished.)

Levels	*Scale Items*	*Clinical Examples*
Level 1	Negative attitude toward self most of the time.	"He is always cutting himself down, no matter how well he does."
Level 2	Negative attitude toward self much of the time.	"If a girl doesn't want to date him, he goes to pieces . . . blames himself a lot."
Level 3	Almost equal in positive and negative attitude toward self.	"One day she can conquer the world; the next she is ready to crawl in a hole and die."
Level 4	Positive attitude toward self much of the time.	"I wish he had more self-confidence, but all in all, he's a pretty good kid . . . makes a real good effort at whatever he undertakes."
Level 5	Positive attitude toward self most of the time.	"Always self-assured . . . will start a conversation with anybody."

Children

Family Interaction: This scale taps the dimension of dependence-independence-interdependence; it is assessing the child's level of functioning in his or her home environment, irrespective of whether the home is the family home, a group home, a foster home, or another kind of living arrangement.

Levels	*Scale Items*	*Clinical Examples*
Level 1	Often must have help with basic needs (for example, feeding, dressing, toilet).	"Refuses to get dressed, even on a school day . . . never learned to tie his shoes."
Level 2	Occasionally needs some help with dressing or feeding.	"She demands attention . . . at times doesn't do things on her own like other kids of her age."
Level 3	Seldom needs help with dressing or feeding. Sometimes helps with family chores when asked.	"It's easier now that he can do more things on his own, but we can't depend on him when we ask him to pick up after himself."
Level 4	Takes care of self and usually helps with family chores when asked.	"If he's in a good mood, he's a joy to have around . . . he usually helps when asked."
Level 5	Takes care of self and willingly helps with family chores.	"Always helps out . . . keeps his room pretty clean . . . takes the garbage out regularly."

Occupation (School): This scale assesses a child's primary occupational role, which is his or her academic performance in comparison to established norms for his or her chronological age. When a child is temporarily out of school due to vacation or sickness, for example, the rating should reflect that child's regular functioning and not the temporary condition he or she is in during the evaluation period (as long as the interviewer is convinced that these circumstances are temporary and not due to the child's behavior or attitude, such as being expelled from school).

Levels	*Scale Items*	*Clinical Examples*
Level 1	Failed all school subjects.	"The teachers say he's not passing anything."
Level 2	Failed more than half school subjects.	"She's only good in math, refuses to work at anything else."

Level 3	Passed more than half school subjects, but not all.	"He has some subjects he does pretty well in, but flunks English every term."
Level 4	Passed all school subjects, but with difficulty.	"He does OK, but seems to have to work harder than the other kids . . . the teacher asked us to give him some extra help at home and it seems to be working."
Level 5	Passed all school subjects with little or no difficulty.	"She's doing well at school . . . and no one ever calls to complain."

Getting Along with Others: This scale is designed to tap the dimension of socialization. It assesses the quality of relationships established with peers outside one's family circle. (Note that this scale does not attempt to differentiate the hostile child from the recluse; both are considered equally unsocialized.)

Levels	*Scale Items*	*Clinical Examples*
Level 1	Always fighting or destructive; or always alone.	"I can't trust him out of my sight for a minute . . . he'll be hitting someone . . . never see him playing nicely with other kids."
Level 2	Seldom able to get along with others without quarreling or being destructive; or is often alone.	"She's getting into fights with neighborhood kids . . . they pick on her . . . prefers to be left alone and read if she doesn't have nice friends."
Level 3	Sometimes quarreling, but seldom destructive; difficulties in making friends.	"He seems to argue a lot with the other kids . . . has few friends . . . always wants his own way."
Level 4	Gets along with others most of the time; has occasional close friends.	"She usually plays with the kid from across the street . . . not many others . . . oh, she has her days, but usually she plays well."

| Level 5 | Gets along with others most of the time; has regular close friends. | "Kids are always coming by to play with him . . . he enjoys seeing his friends at school each day . . . has two really good friends." |

Feelings and Mood: This scale taps the level of affective modulation as indicated by the degree to which feelings are flexibly expressed and adaptively integrated into overall personality functioning. Careful observation is needed of the child's emotional status during the diagnostic interview as well as evaluation of the significant others' reports about the child's feelings in a variety of personal and social situations.

Levels	*Scale Items*	*Clinical Examples*
Level 1	Almost always feels nervous, or depressed, or angry and bitter, or no emotions at all.	"You *never* get a civil word from her . . . she seems to be crying all the time."
Level 2	Often feels nervous, or depressed, or angry and bitter, or hardly shows any emotion for weeks at a time.	"Since his father left, he has just been moping around most of the time."
Level 3	Frequently in a good mood but occasionally feels nervous, or depressed, or angry for days at a time.	"She takes everything so hard, a disappointment can spoil her whole week."
Level 4	Usually in a good mood but occasionally feels nervous, or unhappy, or angry all day.	"He feels fine most of the time . . . well, occasionally he seems to get up on the wrong side and nothing goes right that day for him."
Level 5	In a good mood most of the time, and usually able to be as happy, or sad, or angry as the situation calls for.	"Boy, can she get angry! But it usually passes quickly . . . she has a fine disposition most of the time."

Use of Free Time: This scale is designed to measure the degree to which sublimatory processes have satisfactorily evolved by indicating how free or constricted the child is in his or her use of inner and outer resources for play and enjoyment. In rating the client on this scale, the interviewer should bear in mind that hobbies and recreational activities may satisfactorily be engaged in alone or with other people.

Levels	Scale Items	Clinical Examples
Level 1	Almost no recreational activities or hobbies.	"He has no initiative at all . . . he just sits or lies in his room most of the weekend . . . not interested in anything."
Level 2	Only occasional recreational activities, or repeats the same activity over and over again.	"It drives me mad the way she always expects *me* to find her something to do . . . she ends up watching TV most of the time."
Level 3	Participates in some recreational activities or hobbies.	"Sometimes he plays ball with the other kids . . . he really doesn't have enough friends to do things with."
Level 4	Often participates in recreational activities and hobbies.	"She's in Girl Scouts . . . can't wait for summer camp . . . enjoys going with her friends to movies and picnics."
Level 5	Participates in, as well as creates, variety of own recreational activities and hobbies.	"Likes to be involved in things . . . even on a rainy day, he can always find something enjoyable to do."

Problems: This scale was designed to tap the coping capacity the child can bring to bear on daily problems. At the lowest level of functioning the child is unable to handle even mild problems, hence, he or she experiences severe difficulties most of the time. At the highest level of functioning, the child is able to handle well even severe problems; therefore, he or she is described as having only occasionally mild problems. ("Severe" refers to problems that are incapacitating in important areas, such as school, play, or communication; "moderate" refers to problems that are impairing one's efficiency and/or effectiveness but are not totally incapacitating; "mild" refers to problems that are annoying or inconveniencing but do not incapacitate or interfere with functioning in important areas.)

Levels	Scale Items	Clinical Examples
Level 1	Severe problems most of the time.	"He just doesn't grow up . . . I can't leave him alone for a minute . . . I'm afraid of what he might do . . . he needs constant supervision."
Level 2	Severe problems some of the time or moderate problems continuously.	"Sometimes things really seem to fall apart . . . on those days, I usually keep him home from school."
Level 3	Moderate problems most of the time, or mild problems almost continuously.	"She's usually a handful, but some days are better than others."
Level 4	Occasional moderate problems.	"She can get pretty upset if she doesn't get her way, but if a friend calls or visits, you would think she didn't have a problem in the world!"
Level 5	Occasional mild problems.	"Only once in a while things don't work out well, but some comforting usually puts things right again for her . . . she really manages well."

Attitude toward Self: This scale is designed to tap the dimension of self-esteem in terms of the balance of negative and positive attitudes expressed about the self. Children are rated on the basis of observations in the diagnostic interview, as well as on the basis of reports from significant others about how the child is feeling and acting in a variety of situations (such as with friends, in school, or in sports) and not on the basis of inferential deductions derived from theory. For example, if a truant boy likes himself and has an overall positive attitude, he is to be rated highly on the *Attitude toward Self* scale, even though psychoanalytic theory may suggest that his truancy is indicative of low self-esteem. (Since truancy leads to punishment, the theory might postulate that the child has low self-esteem, which is unconsciously driving him to violate regulations and be punished.)

Levels	Scale Items	Clinical Examples
Level 1	Negative attitude toward self most of the time.	"In school they say he's afraid to try anything new . . . he says he can't do it . . . I guess I see that at home, too."
Level 2	Negative attitude toward self much of the time.	"Even though she is capable, she many times lacks the confidence to tell the teacher she can do the work."
Level 3	Almost equal in positive and negative attitude toward self.	"She is OK when we are alone, but feels like hiding in a corner when in a crowd . . . she suddenly becomes shy and unsure of herself when faced with people she doesn't know well."
Level 4	Positive attitude toward self much of the time.	"Usually willing to try something new . . . feels he'll succeed."
Level 5	Positive attitude toward self most of the time.	"She's a very happy kid . . . interested in trying new things."

Developmentally Disabled

Family Interaction: This scale taps the dimension of dependence-independence-interdependence; it is assessing the client's level of functioning in his or her home environment, irrespective of whether the home is the family home, a group home, a foster home, or another kind of living arrangement.

Levels	Scale Items	Clinical Examples
Level 1	Often must have help with basic needs (for example, feeding, dressing, toilet).	"Unable to dress self, feed self, or take care of toilet needs without supervision and assistance from others."

Level 2	Occasionally needs some help with dressing, feeding, or toilet; able to help others when asked.	"Needs some supervision with dressing, feeding, or toileting; responds to helping others only when prodded."
Level 3	Takes care of self and sometimes helps with home chores.	"Takes care of basic needs with no help from others; sometimes does household chores without having to be reminded."
Level 4	Takes care of self and assumes regularly assigned responsibilities in the home.	"Takes care of own basic needs; performs regularly assigned chores and helps others without having to be asked."
Level 5	Takes care of self and shares responsibilities and planning with others in the home.	"Takes care of own needs and helps others willingly; participates in planning activities in the home."

Occupation (School-Job-Homemaking): This scale taps a person's level of functioning in his or her primary occupational role. When a person is temporarily laid off, or out of the program due to vacation, sick leave, and the like, the rating should reflect that person's regular functioning and not the temporary condition he or she is in during the evaluation period (as long as the interviewer is convinced that these circumstances are temporary and not due to client's behavior or attitude).

Levels	*Scale Items*	*Clinical Examples*
Level 1	Does not participate in planned program (such as special education, day activities, or sheltered workshop) or work.	"Stays at home most of the time . . . doesn't do anything."
Level 2	Occasionally participates in planned program or work (up to 25 percent of the time).	"Goes to a planned program about one day a week . . . doesn't like to participate."

Level 3	Often participates in planned program or work (between 25 percent and 50 percent of the time).	"Goes to a planned program about two days a week" or "Works a couple of days a week on the farm."
Level 4	Usually participates in planned program or work (between 50 percent and 75 percent of the time).	"Usually attends a program three or four days a week" or "Holds a half-time job."
Level 5	Almost always participates in planned program or work (over 75 percent of the time).	"Usually goes to a program five days a week" or "Holds a full-time job."

Getting Along with Others: This scale is designed to tap the dimension of socialization; it assesses the quality of relationships established with people outside one's home (these people may be personal friends, relatives, or family friends). (Note that this scale does not attempt to differentiate the hostile person from the recluse; both are considered equally unsocialized.)

Levels	*Scale Items*	*Clinical Examples*
Level 1	Always fighting or destructive; or always alone.	"Stays by himself almost all the time; when with others, gets easily mad and hits or throws things."
Level 2	Seldom able to get along with others without quarreling or being destructive; or is often alone.	"Has a hard time being around others without quarreling; prefers to stay home."
Level 3	Sometimes quarreling, but seldom destructive; difficulties in making friends.	"Hard to get along with people outside the family."
Level 4	Gets along with others most of the time; has occasional friends.	"Able to get along with people most of the time and has some friends."
Level 5	Gets along with others most of the time; has regular friends.	"Is comfortable being around other people; has regular friends."

Feelings and Mood: This scale taps the level of affective modulation as indicated by the degree to which feelings are flexibly expressed and adaptively integrated into overall personality functioning. Careful observation is needed of the client's emotional status during the diagnostic interview as well as evaluation of the significant others' reports about the client's feelings in a variety of personal and social situation.

Levels	Scale Items	Clinical Examples
Level 1	Almost always feels nervous, or depressed, or angry and bitter, or no emotions at all.	"Does not offer to show any feelings or seems to always be upset."
Level 2	Often feels nervous, or depressed, or angry and bitter, or hardly shows any emotion for weeks at a time.	"Seems to be upset for weeks at a time."
Level 3	Frequently in a good mood but occasionally feels nervous, or depressed, or angry for days at a time.	"Often appears happy, but sometimes seems to get upset for several days."
Level 4	Usually in a good mood but occasionally feels nervous, or unhappy, or angry all day.	"Usually happy, but sometimes has a bad day."
Level 5	In a good mood most of the time, and usually able to be as happy, or sad, or angry as the situation calls for.	"Feels OK most of the time and expresses feelings appropriate to the situation."

Use of Free Time: This scale is designed to measure the degree to which sublimatory processes have satisfactorily evolved by indicating how free or constricted a person is in his or her use of inner and outer resources for play and enjoyment. In rating the client on this scale, the interviewer should bear in mind that hobbies and recreational activities may satisfactorily be engaged in alone or with other people.

Levels	Scale Items	Clinical Examples
Level 1	Almost no recreational activities or hobbies.	"She's home all the time . . . doesn't do anything."

Level 2	Only occasional recreational activities, or repeats the same activity over and over again.	"Watches television all the time."
Level 3	Participates in some recreational activities or hobbies.	"Goes bowling once in a while . . . when invited."
Level 4	Often participates in recreational activities and hobbies.	"Regularly goes to picnics and to the movies with others."
Level 5	Participates in, as well as creates, variety of own recreational activities and hobbies.	"Able to fill his free time himself; enjoys going with others fishing or bowling."

Problems: This scale was designed to tap the coping capacity the person can bring to bear on daily problems. At the lowest level of functioning, the person is unable to handle even mild problems; hence, he or she experiences severe difficulties most of the time. At the highest level of functioning, the individual is able to handle well even severe problems; therefore, he or she is described as having only occasionally mild problems. ("Severe" refers to problems that are incapacitating in important areas, such as homemaking, work, or communication; "moderate" refers to problems that are impairing one's efficiency and/or effectiveness but are not totally incapacitating; "mild" refers to problems that are annoying or inconveniencing but do not incapacitate or interfere with a person's functioning in important areas in their lives.)

Levels	*Scale Items*	*Clinical Examples*
Level 1	Severe problems most of the time.	"Refuses to talk to anyone or do anything."
Level 2	Severe problems some of the time or moderate problems continuously.	"Often refuses to attend planned programs."
Level 3	Moderate problems most of time, or mild problems almost continuously.	"Attends planned programs but refuses to learn new things."
Level 4	Occasional moderate problems.	"Overall, gets along; responds to encouragement from others."

| Level 5 | Occasional mild problems. | "Seems to be able to work things out even when there are problems." |

Attitude toward Self: This scale is designed to tap the dimension of self-esteem in terms of the balance of negative and positive attitudes expressed about the self. Clients are rated on the basis of observations in the diagnostic interview as well as on the basis of reports from significant others about how the client is feeling and acting in a variety of situations (for example, client feels deserving-undeserving; hopeful-hopeless; assertive-resigned; mixes-isolated; inferior-competent at what he or she is doing).

Levels	*Scale Items*	*Clinical Examples*
Level 1	Negative attitude toward self most of the time.	"Feels nobody likes him."
Level 2	Negative attitude toward self much of the time.	"Doesn't like to try, because things have never worked before."
Level 3	Almost equal in positive and negative attitude toward self.	"Enjoys himself in the program but hates weekends."
Level 4	Positive attitude toward self much of the time.	"Appears to be adjusting well."
Level 5	Positive attitude toward self most of the time.	"Is happy most of the time with what he does."

Appendix B
Consumer Satisfaction
Questionnaire Studies

A. Introduction
B. Return Rate of CSQ
C. Frequency Distribution of Client Responses to the CSQ
D. Relationship of CSQ to Progress Evaluation Scale Ratings

The consumer satisfaction questionnaire (CSQ) studies used a modified version of a questionnaire developed by the Department of Psychiatry, University of Cincinnati. The revised questionnaire consists of thirteen items displayed on one page, with an invitation for additional client comments at the end of the questionnaire. (See figure B–1.) The directions on the CSQ instruct clients to check one of the statements following each question, for the first nine items. The items that follow inquire whether clients were treated with medication for the condition for which they have requested services and whether the medication was prescribed through the mental-health center. Clients are also asked whether they found the medication suitable and in the right amount. Additionally clients are asked whether they think that the fees charged for center services were justifiable.

The questionnaire is mailed, together with the PES form and a cover letter, to all community mental-health center clients whose records are closed. The results from the returned questionnaires are scored by a clerical person by superimposing a template on the filled-out questionnaire; the template converts client-marked responses into numerical values. The value of 1 is keyed to the most negative response alternative (for example, the client got worse as a result of service), while 5 or 6 is keyed to the most positive alternatives. It takes two to three minutes to score the questionnaire. The numerical values of the alternatives to each question are marked on the attached sample.

If clients add comments to their CSQ responses (about 50 percent do), these are brought to the attention of their therapists by the transcribing secretary. Serious complaints from clients on the questionnaire are brought to the attention of the agency director; the director reviews these complaints with therapists, following established agency procedures for reviewing patient complaints.

Return Rate of CSQ

A survey of the literature conducted by Albers (1977) revealed that the return rate for consumer satisfaction questionnaires usually does not exceed 30 percent. In a series of six studies, we undertook to explore the impact of a number of different administration procedures on return rate.

In the first study, 624 patients were mailed the CSQ with a cover letter, three to six months after the last face-to-face interview with the mental-health center staff. In this study patients' names were written on top of the questionnaires. Return rate was 26 percent.

Under the second condition, involving 111 clients, the space earmarked for the client's name was crossed out. For emphasis, clients were asked in the cover letter not to mark any personally identifying formation on the CSQ. Return rate for this group was 27 percent.

The third sample consisted of 299 clients; this time, the space earmarked for the client's name was left unmarked. In the cover letter clients were informed that they could either write their name on top of the questionnaires or leave the space for name blank. Of those who returned the CSQ, 81.9 percent chose to write their names in. Overall return rate under these instructions was 24 percent.

In the fourth study the questionnaires were mailed to 511 clients; this was followed up with an attempt to contact each client by telephone four or five days later. Whenever telephone contact was established, the clients were asked whether they received our questionnaire and whether they had any difficulty filling it out; then they were urged to mail it in that day or the following day. Additionally patients were informed over the telephone that if they could not take the questionnaire to a mail box, we could send someone from the center to their home to pick it up. Results indicate that 41 percent of all patients were successfully contacted by telephone; of this group, 34 percent said they would return the questionnaire by mail and did so; 48 percent said they would return the questionnaire but have not done so; 8 percent said they did not want to fill out the questionnaire; and another 10 percent were noncommittal, making such statements as, "I need to think it over." Of the patients whom we could not reach by telephone (59 percent), 13 percent did not have telephones, 20 percent had their telephones disconnected, 29 percent recently moved, and another 29 percent could not be reached after three telephone calls (morning, afternoon, and evening) over a two-day period. In summary, of the 511 questionnaires mailed, 25 percent were filled out and returned, 11 percent were returned unopened due to no forwarding address, and 64 percent were not returned.

Figure B–1 Shiawassee County Community Mental Health Services Board Consumer Satisfaction Questionnaire

Name_____Date_____

Please check *one* answer after each of the following questions:

1. How much did you benefit from the service you received at the Mental Health Center?

   1 _____ Not at all
   2 _____ Very little
   3 _____ To some extent
   4 _____ A fair amount
   5 _____ A great deal

2. To what extent have your problems or symptoms that brought you to the Center changed as a result of treatment or services rendered?

   1 _____ Got worse
   2 _____ Not at all improved
   3 _____ Somewhat improved
   4 _____ Considerably improved
   5 _____ Very greatly improved
   6 _____ Completely gone

3. On the whole, how well do you feel you are getting along now?

   5 _____ Very well
   4 _____ Fairly well
   3 _____ Neither well nor poorly
   2 _____ Fairly poorly
   1 _____ Very poorly

4. How much do you feel you have changed as a result of being served by the Center?

   5 _____ A great deal
   4 _____ A fair amount
   3 _____ Somewhat
   2 _____ Very little
   1 _____ Not at all

5. Did your therapist really understand your problems?

   5 _____ Completely
   4 _____ Quite well
   3 _____ To some extent
   2 _____ Very little
   1 _____ Not at all

6. Did you get as many appointments at the Center as you needed?

   5 _____ Just what I needed
   4 _____ About right
   3 _____ Barely enough
   2 _____ Somewhat too few
   1 _____ Much too few

7. How much further service do you feel you need now?

   5 _____ No need at all
   4 _____ Slight need
   3 _____ Could use more
   2 _____ Considerable need
   1 _____ Very great need

8. Everything considered, how satisfied are you with the results of our services?

   1 _____ Very dissatisfied
   2 _____ Moderately dissatisfied
   3 _____ Fairly satisfied
   4 _____ Moderately satisfied
   5 _____ Very satisfied

9. Would you recommend the Mental Health Center to a close friend with emotional problems?

   1 _____ Would advise against it
   2 _____ Would not recommend it
   3 _____ Would recommend it but with some reservations
   4 _____ Would mildly recommend it
   5 _____ Would strongly recommend it

10. Were the problems or symptoms for which you received service at the Mental Health Center also treated with medication? (Read all answers before marking one or more responses.)

   _____ Prescribed at Mental Health Center
   _____ Prescribed by another physician
   _____ Obtained without prescription
   _____ No medication

11. Did it seem to be the kind of medication you needed? (Mark one if relevant)

   _____ Yes
   _____ Uncertain
   _____ No

12. Did the medication seem to be in the right amount? (Mark one if relevant)

   _____ Not enough
   _____ Just about right
   _____ Too much

13. Did you feel that the fee set for you at the Mental Health Center was justifiable?

   _____ Yes
   _____ No (Too high)
   _____ No (Too low)

We would appreciate receiving any additional comments you may have regarding our services. Please use more paper if needed. Thank you for your cooperation.

Note: Scoring key is marked in front of responses for questions 1 through 9. Permission is hereby granted to agencies and individuals to reproduce the Consumer Satisfaction Questionnaire for professional use.

The fifth study entailed mailing a reminder a week after the original mailing of the CSQ and an attempted telephone call a week later, if there was no reply to our written reminder. The return rate under this condition was 26 percent.

The sixth study in this series entailed a random assignment of a group of 75 adult clients, drawn in about equal number from eight center therapists, to three conditions. One group of 25 clients was mailed a cover letter with the CSQ and one dollar; a second group was mailed the letter and was promised that one dollar would be forthcoming when we received the filled-out questionnaire; the third group was mailed the questionnaire with the same letter as the other two groups but without any reference to money. Results showed that the group that was mailed the one dollar responded at a much higher rate than either of the other two groups. Of the 25 clients who were mailed one dollar, 44 percent returned the filled-out CSQ (two envelopes were returned unopened due to lack of a forwarding address); of the 25 clients who were promised one dollar if they returned the filled-out questionnaire, 20 percent did so (one CSQ could not be delivered); of the 25 clients who received the regular cover letter with no mention of money, 24 percent returned the questionnaire (one envelope could not be delivered). It appears that mailing one dollar with the CSQ can almost double the return rate. Other approaches to improve return rate of CSQ need to be explored. One possibility is the use of originally typed letters, which can be done easily with word processors; cover letters might be signed by clients' primary therapists.

Frequency Distribution of Client Responses to the CSQ

The tabulation of client responses in table B–1 displays in percentages the level of satisfaction with various aspects of mental-health services in six different mailings. The first four mailings correspond to the first four studies described previously. The last two mailings are the responses of clients in more-recent studies in which their names were written on the body of the questionnaire. Level of satisfaction is regularly analyzed for various programs, with results shared continuously with the staff. Improvement of satisfaction in some categories was noted in later mailings.

Relationship of CSQ to Progress Evaluation Scale Ratings

Fifty-eight adult women and 44 men who were treated at the Shiawassee County Mental Health Center filled out both the CSQ and the PES. They

Table B–1
Summary of Results from Six Mailings of Consumer Satisfaction Questionnaire

	Mailings					
	1	2	3	4	5	6
Number mailed	624	111	299	511	263	84
Percentage returned	26	27	24	25	34	36
1. How much did you benefit from the service you received at the mental-health center?						
Not at all and very little	17%	17%	21%	23%	12%	15%
To some extent	10	30	16	19	17	27
A fair amount and a great deal	64	53	63	58	71	58
2. To what extent have your problems or symptoms that brought you to the center changed as a result of treatment or services rendered?						
Got worse and not at all improved	16	20	18	20	9	13
Somewhat improved	31	30	32	33	26	34
Considerably improved and very greatly improved and completely gone	53	30	50	47	65	53
3. On the whole, how well do you feel you are getting along now?						
Very well and fairly well	76	90	75	71	78	69
Neither well nor poorly	18	7	15	16	19	19
Fairly poorly and very poorly	6	3	10	13	3	12
4. How much do you feel you have changed as a result of being served by the center?						
A great deal and a fair amount	59	61	54	46	56	40
Somewhat	20	19	19	27	29	27
Very little and not at all	21	20	27	27	15	33
5. Did your therapist really understand your problems?						
Completely and quite well	65	60	68	58	79	80
To some extent	21	23	16	26	17	17
Very little and not at all	14	17	16	16	4	3

Table B-1 continued

	Number	Percentage				
6. Did you get as many appointments at the center as you needed?						
Just what I needed and about right	91	77	73	84	82	84
Barely enough	4	10	13	2	7	2
Somewhat too few and much too few	5	13	14	14	11	14
7. How much further service do you feel you need now?						
No need at all and slight need	69	59	63	66	60	68
Could use more	23	28	22	19	26	16
Considerable need and very great need	8	13	15	15	14	16
8. Everything considered, how satisfied are you with the results of our services?						
Very dissatisfied and moderately dissatisfied	19	27	28	15	14	10
Fairly satisfied	19	23	14	27	23	10
Moderately satisfied and very satisfied	62	50	58	58	63	80
9. Were the problems or symptoms for which you received service at the mental-health center also treated with medication?						
Prescribed at mental-health center	23	32	22	13	20	21
Prescribed by another physician	18	12	15	16	14	28
Obtained without prescription	1	6	3	3	1	0
No medication	58	50	60	68	65	51
10. Did it seem to be the kind of medication you needed?						
Yes	55	33⅓	32	66	60	65
Uncertain	26	33⅓	36	24	22	29
No	19	33⅓	32	10	18	6
11. Did it seem to be the right amount?						
Not enough	14	16	20	15	11	6
Just about right	72	46	65	85	66	88
Too much	14	38	15	0	23	6

12. Would you recommend the mental-health center to a close friend with emotional problems?

Would advise against it and would not recommend it	8	6	8	6	7	0
Would recommend it but with some reservations	16	18	9	11	7	6
Would mildly recommend it and would strongly recommend it	76	76	83	83	86	94

13. Did you feel that the fee set for you at the mental-health center was justifiable?

Yes	95	93	95	93	97	97
No (too high)	3	7	4	4	3	0
No (too low)	1	0	1	3	0	3

14. If a follow-up appointment with your therapist is scheduled in three months, would you be willing to come? (There will be no charge.)

Yes	78	81	82	85	88	81
No	22	19	18	15	12	19

15. We would appreciate receiving any additional comments you may have regarding our services. Please use more paper if needed.

Comments	52	57	53	51	55	55
No comments	48	43	47	49	44	45

Table B–2
Means, Standard Deviations, and Intercorrelations of Items on Consumer Satisfaction Questionnaire for Samples of Male and Female Psychiatric Outpatients

	$\bar{X}$	sd	2	3	4	5	6	7	8	9	Sum Score
Males											
1 Benefit from service	3.66	1.24	76	48	71	74	49	−11	76	65	87
2 Problems changed as result of treatment	3.70	1.23		65	69	55	48	23	65	51	87
3 Getting along now	3.73	1.17			59	47	50	40	54	40	75
4 Personal change	3.16	1.31				55	41	06	68	62	83
5 Therapist understanding	3.64	1.08					46	−28	72	63	74
6 Sufficient appointments	4.10	1.01						31	39	13	63
7 Present need for services	3.74	1.00							−03	−22	19
8 Satisfied with results	3.89	1.32								67	84
9 Would recommend MHC	4.27	1.06									69
10 Sum score	34.19	7.52									
Females											
1 Benefit from service	3.77	1.29	72	24	70	72	36	18	73	70	86
2 Problems changed as result of treatment	3.68	1.09		46	63	63	17	46	56	52	81
3 Getting along now	4.05	.85			33	22	03	72	06	12	47
4 Personal change	3.54	1.17				56	29	24	54	59	78
5 Therapist understanding	3.77	1.09					24	23	73	77	83
6 Sufficient appointments	4.11	1.08						16	28	32	45
7 Present need for services	3.91	1.17							13	06	47
8 Satisfied with results	3.72	1.51								75	78
9 Would recommend MHC	4.28	1.19									77
10 Sum score	34.98	7.38									

Note: Decimal points for correlations are omitted.

Table B–3

Correlations between Consumer Satisfaction Questionnaire Items and Age, Education, Number of Sessions, and PES Closing-Status Scores, for Females (N = 58)

Variable		1	2	3	4	5	6	7	8	9	Total
							CSQ Items				
Age		25	26*	22	16	22	26	13	18	12	30*
Education		-14	-12	-20	-31*	-16	-18	00	-16	-33*	-30*
Number of sessions		02	01	-22	-03	-04	09	-04	-03	13	-03
Closing status											
Family Interaction	Therapist	32*	29*	29*	25	13	11	25	18	20	29*
	Patient	21	38**	55**	25	23	11	57**	10	04	34*
Occupation	Therapist	28*	15	13	35**	11	25	08	07	14	28**
	Patient	16	27*	33*	21	29*	11	34**	25	20	37**
Getting Along	Therapist	30*	15	04	39**	11	14	00	20	27*	31*
with Others	Patient	14	31*	30*	28*	24	20	45**	09	21	34*
Feelings and Mood	Therapist	17	20	21	23	-02	24	15	15	14	27
	Patient	14	43**	65**	32*	19	07	74**	08	07	43**
Use of Free Time	Therapist	12	07	00	18	-05	02	-13	00	05	09
	Patient	-03	12	33*	23	15	05	38**	-04	08	26
Problems	Therapist	25	31*	14	36**	11	18	21	18	14*	35**
	Patient	32*	38**	55**	50**	34**	30*	69**	33*	33*	61**
Attitude toward Self	Therapist	19	24	14	29*	04	20	17	09	07	24
	Patient	17	29*	59**	28*	20	11	59**	10	18	42**

Note: Decimals are omitted.

*$p < 0.05$.
**$p < 0.01$.

Table B–4
Correlations between Consumer Satisfaction Questionnaire Items and Age, Education, Number of Sessions, and PES Closing-Status Scores, for Males (N = 44)

		CSQ Items									
Variable		*1*	*2*	*3*	*4*	*5*	*6*	*7*	*8*	*9*	*Total*
Age		-06	-07	-25	01	-05	05	-15	-15	10	-02
Education		-04	05	18	07	-23	16	25	-09	-08	01
Number of sessions		28	41**	28	25	32*	30	-08	09	11	29
Closing status											
Family Interaction	Therapist	42**	44**	40**	44**	52**	22	-02	45**	61**	51**
	Patient	37*	34*	39**	22	17	28	21	15	01	29
Occupation	Therapist	38**	37*	46**	57**	34*	46**	24	37*	31*	50**
	Patient	24	31*	46**	35*	18	19	32*	24	07	28
Getting Along with Others	Therapist	37*	24	23	33*	37*	35*	-04	27	22	33*
	Patient	30*	32*	50**	30*	35*	24	27	27	27	35*
Feelings and Mood	Therapist	58**	57**	50**	57**	52**	34*	01	45**	38**	60**
	Patient	24	39*	52**	21	20	22	35*	22	03	35*
Use of Free Time	Therapist	30*	38*	35*	47**	31*	23	08	28	18	41**
	Patient	17	35*	43*	32*	07	10	36*	14	16	27
Problems	Therapist	44**	54**	41**	39**	49**	34*	09	32*	28	52**
	Patient	43**	55**	67**	39**	39**	45**	39**	34*	16	55**
Attitude toward Self	Therapist	44**	58**	58**	46**	39**	45**	17	39**	15	54**
	Patient	20	36*	30*	43**	11	26	39**	26	02	31*

Note: Decimals are omitted.
*$p < 0.05$.
**$p < 0.01$

were also rated by their therapists on the PES. The means and standard deviations for initial status, goals, and closing status by therapists and patients have been presented in tables 2–21 and 2–22. Here we present only data on the CSQ and its relation to the PES ratings of client and therapist.

Table B–2 shows the intercorrelations of the first nine items of the CSQ, as well as the means and standard deviations for each item. With the exception of a few relationships, most items are positively correlated, indicating that a common factor permeates the first nine questions in the questionnaire. The three negative correlations in the male sample are of some interest. "Need for services at termination" is negatively correlated $(r = -0.28)$ with "therapists' understanding" of their patients' problems; "Need for services at termination" is negatively correlated $(r = -0.22)$ with the likelihood of "Recommending mental-health services" to other people with emotional problems; and "Need for services at termination" is negatively correlated $(r = -0.11)$ with the "Amount of benefit derived from therapy." These correlations are all low positive for the female sample. Further research is required to understand this sex difference in satisfaction with services. At least for men, this finding suggests that "Need for services" may not be linearly related to satisfaction since the person who feels helped may now be willing to acknowledge that further help could be useful.

Tables B–3 and B–4 present the correlations for females and males, respectively, between the first nine CSQ items and age, education, number of sessions seen, and PES closing-status scores. Overall, age is positively correlated $(r = 0.30)$ with client satisfaction with therapy, while education is negatively correlated $(r = -0.30)$. The underlying reasons for this finding need further exploration. Number of sessions, on the other hand, is not related to satisfaction with services $(r = -0.03)$. Most correlations between PES closing ratings and the CSQ sum score are significant and all are positive, whether the ratings were made by the therapist or the patient. However, the correlations between therapist ratings and the CSQ tend to be higher for the males, whereas correlations between self-ratings and the CSQ are higher for the females. These data tend to support the use of consumer satisfaction questionnaires as one indication of treatment outcome.

Appendix C
Progress Evaluation
Scale Forms

Although the PES forms appearing in this appendix are copyrighted, permission is hereby granted to agencies and individuals to reproduce them for professional use.

Adult PES Form 1: Present Functioning

Screening _____
Initial _____
Reeval. No. _____
Closing _____

Client _____ CR TD DX UA OT
M/F/O—Sig. Other _____ CR TD DX UA OT
Therapist _____

Name _____

Date _____

Case # _____

INSTRUCTIONS—1

Please circle one statement in each column that describes best how you were in the last two weeks.

Family Interaction	Occupation (School, Job or Homemaking)	Getting Along with Others	Feelings and Mood	Use of Free Time	Problems	Attitude toward Self
Often must have help with basic needs (for example, feeding, dressing, toilet).	Does not hold job, or care for home, or go to school.	Always fighting or destructive; or always alone.	Almost always feels nervous, or depressed, or angry and bitter, or no emotions at all.	Almost no recreational activities or hobbies.	Severe problems most of the time.	Negative attitude toward self most of the time.
Takes care of own basic needs but must have help with everyday plans and activities.	Seldom holds job, or attends classes, or cares for home.	Seldom able to get along with others without quarreling or being destructive; or is often alone.	Often feels nervous, or depressed, or angry and bitter, or hardly shows any emotion for weeks at a time.	Only occasional recreational activities, or repeats the same activity over and over again.	Severe problems some of the time or moderate problems continuously.	Negative attitude toward self much of time.

Makes own plans but without considering the needs of other family members.	Sometimes holds job, or attends some classes, or does limited housework.	Sometimes quarreling, but seldom destructive difficulties in making friends.	Frequently in a good mood but occasionally feels nervous, or depressed, or angry for days at a time.	Participates in some recreational activities or hobbies.	Moderate problems most of time, or mild problems almost continuously.	Almost equal in positive and negative attitude toward self.
Tries to consider everyone's needs but somehow decisions and actions do not work well for everybody in the family.	Holds regular job, or classes, or does housework (or some combination of these), but with difficulty.	Gets along with others most of the time; has occasional close friends.	Usually in a good mood, but occasionally feels nervous, or unhappy, or angry all day.	Often participates in recreational activities and hobbies.	Occasional moderate problems.	Positive attitude toward self much of the time.
Usually plans and acts so that own needs as well as needs of others in the family are considered.	Holds regular job, or attends classes, or does housework (or some combination of these) with little or no difficulty.	Gets along with others most of the time; has regular close friends.	In a good mood most of the time, and usually able to be as happy, or sad, or angry as the situation calls for.	Participates in, as well as creates, variety of own recreational activities and hobbies for self and others.	Occasional mild problems.	Positive attitude toward self most of the time.

Comments:

Adult PES Form 2: Goals

Screening _____
Initial _____
Reeval. No. _____
Closing _____

     Client _____ CR TD DX UA OT
M/F/O—Sig. Other _____ CR TD DX UA OT
    Therapist _____

Date _____

Name _____   Case # _____

INSTRUCTIONS—2
Please circle one statement in each column that describes best how you expect to be in _____ months.

Family Interaction	Occupation (School, Job or Homemaking)	Getting Along with Others	Feelings and Mood	Use of Free Time	Problems	Attitude toward Self
Often must have help with basic needs (for example, feeding, dressing, toilet).	Does not hold job, or care for home, or go to school.	Always fighting or destructive; or always alone.	Almost always feels nervous, or depressed, or angry and bitter, or no emotions at all.	Almost no recreational activities or hobbies.	Severe problems most of the time.	Negative attitude toward self most of the time.
Takes care of own basic needs but must have help with everyday plans and activities.	Seldom holds job, or attends classes, or cares for home.	Seldom able to get along with others without quarreling or being destructive; or is often alone.	Often feels nervous, or depressed, or angry and bitter, or hardly shows any emotion for weeks at a time.	Only occasional recreational activities, or repeats the same activity over and over again.	Severe problems some of the time or moderate problems continuously.	Negative attitude toward self much of time.

Makes own plans but without considering the needs of other family members.	Sometimes holds job, or attends some classes, or does limited housework.	Sometimes quarreling, but seldom destructive, in making friends.	Frequently in a good mood but occasionally feels nervous, or depressed, or angry for days at a time.	Participates in some recreational activities or hobbies.	Moderate problems most of time, or mild problems almost continuously.	Almost equal in positive and negative attitude toward self.
Tries to consider everyone's needs but somehow decisions and actions do not work well for everybody in the family.	Holds regular job, or classes, or does housework (or some combination of these), but with difficulty.	Gets along with others most of the time; has occasional close friends.	Usually in a good mood, but occasionally feels nervous, or unhappy, or angry all day.	Often participates in recreational activities and hobbies.	Occasional moderate problems.	Positive attitude toward self much of the time.
Usually plans and acts so that own needs as well as needs of others in the family are considered.	Holds regular job, or attends classes, or does housework (or some combination of these) with little or no difficulty.	Gets along with others most of the time; has regular close friends.	In a good mood most of the time, and usually able to be as happy, or sad, or angry as the situation calls for.	Participates in, as well as creates, variety of own recreational activities and hobbies for self and others.	Occasional mild problems.	Positive attitude toward self most of the time.

Comments:

Adolescents' PES Form 1: Present Functioning

Screening _____
Initial _____
Reeval. No. _____
Closing _____

M/F/O—Sig. Other

Client _____ CR TD DX UA OT
Other _____ CR TD DX UA OT
Therapist _____

Date _____

Case # _____

Name _____

INSTRUCTIONS—1
Please circle one statement in each column that describes best how you were in the last two weeks.

Family Interaction	Occupation (School, Job or Homemaking)	Getting Along with Others	Feelings and Mood	Use of Free Time	Problems	Attitude toward Self
Often must have help with basic needs (for example, feeding, dressing, toilet).	Expelled from school, or dropped out of school, and holds no job.	Always fighting or destructive; or always alone.	Almost always feels nervous, or depressed, or angry and bitter, or no emotions at all.	Almost no recreational activities or hobbies.	Severe problems most of the time.	Negative attitude toward self most of the time.
Takes care of own basic needs but must have help with everyday plans and activities.	Often skips school, or fails most subjects, or seldom holds job.	Seldom able to get along with others without quarreling or being destructive; or is often alone.	Often feels nervous, or depressed, or angry and bitter, or hardly shows any emotion for weeks at a time.	Only occasional recreational activities, or repeats the same activity over and over again.	Severe problems some of the time or moderate problems continuously.	Negative attitude toward self much of the time.

Makes own plans but without considering the needs of other family members.	Some school skipping, but passes most subjects, or sometimes holds job.	Sometimes quarreling, but seldom destructive; difficulties in making friends.	Frequently in a good mood but occasionally feels nervous, or depressed, or angry for days at a time.	Participates in some recreational activities or hobbies.	Moderate problems most of time, or mild problems almost continuously.	Almost equal in positive and negative attitude toward self.
Tries to consider everyone's needs but somehow decisions and actions do not work well for everybody in the family.	Regular school attendance and passes all subjects, or holds regular job (or some combination of these), but with difficulty.	Gets along with others most of the time; has occasional close friends.	Usually in a good mood, but occasionally feels nervous, or unhappy, or angry all day.	Often participates in recreational activities and hobbies.	Occasional moderate problems.	Positive attitude toward self much of the time.
Usually plans and acts so that own needs as well as needs of others in the family are considered.	Regular school attendance and passes all subjects, or holds regular job (or some combination of these) with little or no difficulty.	Gets along with others most of the time; has regular close friends.	In a good mood most of the time, and usually able to be as happy, or sad, or angry as the situation calls for.	Participates in, as well as creates, variety of own recreational activities and hobbies.	Occasional mild problems.	Positive attitude toward self most of the time.

Comments: _____

Adolescents' PES Form 2: Goals

Screening _____
Initial _____
Reeval. No. _____
Closing _____

Client _____ CR TD DX UA OT
M/F/O—Sig. Other _____ CR TD DX UA OT
Therapist _____

Date _____

Case # _____

INSTRUCTIONS—2

Please circle one statement in each column that describes best how you expect to be in _____ months.

Name _____

Family Interaction	Occupation (School, Job or Homemaking)	Getting Along with Others	Feelings and Mood	Use of Free Time	Problems	Attitude toward Self
Often must have help with basic needs (for example, feeding, dressing, toilet).	Expelled from school, or dropped out of school, and holds no job.	Always fighting or destructive; or always alone.	Almost always feels nervous, or depressed, or angry and bitter, or no emotions at all.	Almost no recreational activities or hobbies.	Severe problems most of the time.	Negative attitude toward self most of the time.
Takes care of own basic needs but must have help with everyday plans and activities.	Often skips school, or fails most subjects, or seldom holds job.	Seldom able to get along with others without quarreling or being destructive; or is often alone.	Often feels nervous, or depressed, or angry and bitter, or hardly shows any emotion for weeks at a time.	Only occasional recreational activities, or repeats the same activity over and over again.	Severe problems some of the time or moderate problems continuously.	Negative attitude toward self much of the time.

Makes own plans but without considering the needs of other family members.	Some school skipping, but passes most subjects, or sometimes holds job.	Sometimes quarreling, but seldom destructive; difficulties in making friends.	Frequently in a good mood but occasionally feels nervous, or depressed, or angry for days at a time.	Participates in some recreational activities or hobbies.	Moderate problems most of time, or mild problems almost continuously.	Almost equal in positive and negative attitude toward self.
Tries to consider everyone's needs but somehow decisions and actions do not work well for everybody in the family.	Regular school attendance and passes all subjects, or holds regular job (or some combination of these), but with difficulty.	Gets along with others most of the time; has occasional close friends.	Usually in a good mood, but occasionally feels nervous, or unhappy, or angry all day.	Often participates in recreational activities and hobbies.	Occasional moderate problems.	Positive attitude toward self much of the time.
Usually plans and acts so that own needs as well as needs of others in the family are considered.	Regular school attendance and passes all subjects, or holds regular job (or some combination of these) with little or no difficulty.	Gets along with others most of the time; has regular close friends.	In a good mood most of the time, and usually able to be as happy, or sad, or angry as the situation calls for.	Participates in, as well as creates, variety of own recreational activities and hobbies.	Occasional mild problems.	Positive attitude toward self most of the time.

Comments: _____

Children's PES Form 1: Present Functioning

Screening _____
Initial _____
Reeval. No. _____
Closing _____

Client _____ CR TD DX UA OT
M/F/O—Sig. Other _____ CR TD DX UA OT
Therapist _____

Date _____

Case # _____

Name _____

INSTRUCTIONS—1
Please circle one statement in each column that describes best how you were in the last two weeks.

Family Interaction	Occupation (School, Job or Homemaking)	Getting Along with Others	Feelings and Mood	Use of Free Time	Problems	Attitude toward Self
Often must have help with basic needs (for example, feeding, dressing, toilet).	Failed all school subjects.	Always fighting or destructive; or always alone.	Almost always feels nervous, or depressed, or angry and bitter, or no emotions at all.	Almost no recreational activities or hobbies.	Severe problems most of the time.	Negative attitude toward self most of the time.
Occasionally needs some help with dressing or feeding.	Failed more than half school subjects.	Seldom able to get along with others without quarreling or being destructive; or is often alone.	Often feels nervous, or depressed, or angry and bitter, or hardly shows any emotion for weeks at a time.	Only occasional recreational activities, or repeats the same activity over and over again.	Severe problems some of the time or moderate problems continuously.	Negative attitude toward self much of the time.

Seldom needs help with dressing or feeding. Sometimes helps with family chores when asked.	Passed more than half school subjects, but not all.	Sometimes quarreling, but seldom destructive; difficulties in making friends.	Frequently in a good mood but occasionally feels nervous, or depressed, or angry for days at a time.	Participates in some recreational activities or hobbies.	Moderate problems most of time, or mild problems almost continuously.	Almost equal in positive and negative attitude toward self.
Takes care of self and usually helps with family chores when asked.	Passed all school subjects, but with difficulty.	Gets along with others most of the time; has occasional close friends.	Usually in a good mood, but occasionally feels nervous, or unhappy, or angry all day.	Often participates in recreational activities and hobbies.	Occasional moderate problems.	Positive attitude toward self much of the time.
Takes care of self and willingly helps with family chores.	Passed all school subjects with no or little difficulty.	Gets along with others most of the time; has regular close friends.	In a good mood most of the time, and usually able to be as happy, or sad, or angry as the situation calls for.	Participates in, as well as creates, variety of own recreational activities and hobbies.	Occasional mild problems.	Positive attitude toward self most of the time.

Comments:

Children's PES Form 2: Goals

Screening _____
Initial _____
Reeval. No. _____
Closing _____

M/F/O—Sig. Other

Client _____ CR TD DX UA OT
Other _____ CR TD DX UA OT
Therapist _____

Date _____

Case # _____

Name _____

INSTRUCTIONS—2
Please circle one statement in each column that describes best how you expect to be in _____ months.

Family Interaction	Occupation (School, Job or Homemaking)	Getting Along with Others	Feelings and Mood	Use of Free Time	Problems	Attitude toward Self
Often must have help with basic needs (for example, feeding, dressing, toilet).	Failed all school subjects.	Always fighting or destructive; or always alone.	Almost always feels nervous, or depressed, or angry and bitter, or no emotions at all.	Almost no recreational activities or hobbies.	Severe problems most of the time.	Negative attitude toward self most of the time.
Occasionally needs some help with dressing or feeding.	Failed more than half school subjects.	Seldom able to get along with others without quarreling or being destructive; or is often alone.	Often feels nervous, or depressed, or angry and bitter, or hardly shows any emotion for weeks at a time.	Only occasional recreational activities, or repeats the same activity over and over again.	Severe problems some of the time or moderate problems continuously.	Negative attitude toward self much of the time.

Seldom needs help with dressing or feeding. Sometimes helps with family chores when asked.	Passed more than half school subjects, but not all.	Sometimes quarreling, but seldom destructive; difficulties in making friends.	Frequently in a good mood but occasionally feels nervous, or depressed, or angry for days at a time.	Participates in some recreational activities or hobbies.	Moderate problems most of time, or mild problems almost continuously.	Almost equal in positive and negative attitude toward self.
Takes care of self and usually helps with family chores when asked.	Passed all school subjects, but with difficulty.	Gets along with others most of the time; has occasional close friends.	Usually in a good mood, but occasionally feels nervous, or unhappy, or angry all day.	Often participates in recreational activities and hobbies.	Occasional moderate problems.	Positive attitude toward self much of the time.
Takes care of self and willingly helps with family chores.	Passed all school subjects with no or little difficulty.	Gets along with others most of the time; has regular close friends.	In a good mood most of the time, and usually able to be as happy, or sad, or angry as the situation calls for.	Participates in, as well as creates, variety of own recreational activities and hobbies.	Occasional mild problems.	Positive attitude toward self most of the time.

Comments: _____

Developmentally Disabled PES Form 1: Present Functioning

Screening _____
Initial _____
Reeval. No. _____
Closing _____

Client _____ CR TD DX UA OT
M/F/O—Sig. Other _____ CR TD DX UA OT
Therapist _____

Date _____

Case # _____

Name _____

INSTRUCTIONS—1

Please circle one statement in each column that describes best how you were in the last two weeks.

Family Interaction	Occupation (School, Job or Homemaking)	Getting Along with Others	Feelings and Mood	Use of Free Time	Problems	Attitude toward Self
Often must have help with basic needs (for example, feeding, dressing, toilet).	Does not participate in planned program such as Spec. Ed., Day Activities, or Sheltered Workshop) or work.	Always fighting or destructive; or always alone.	Almost always feels nervous, or depressed, or angry and bitter, or no emotions at all.	Almost no recreational activities or hobbies.	Severe problems most of the time.	Negative attitude toward self most of the time.
Occasionally needs some help with dressing, feeding, or toilet; able to help others when asked.	Is occasionally participating in planned program or work (up to 25% of the time).	Seldom able to get along with others without quarreling or being destructive; or is often alone.	Often feels nervous, or depressed, or angry and bitter, or hardly shows any emotion for weeks at a time.	Only occasional recreational activities, or repeats the same activity over and again.	Severe problems some of the time or moderate problems continuously.	Negative attitude toward self much of the time.

Takes care of self and sometimes helps with home chores.	Takes care of self and assumes regularly assigned responsibilities in the home.	Takes care of self and shares responsibilities and planning with others in the home.
Often participates in planned program or work (between 25% and 50% of the time).	Usually participates in planned program or work (between 50% and 75% of the time).	Almost always participates in planned program or work (over 75% of the time).
Sometimes quarreling, but seldom destructive; difficulties in making friends.	Gets along with others most of the time; has occasional friends.	Gets along with others most of the time; has regular friends.
Frequently in a good mood but occasionally feels nervous, or depressed, or angry for days at a time.	Usually in a good mood, but occasionally feels nervous, or unhappy, or angry all day.	In a good mood most of the time, and usually able to be as happy, or sad, or angry as the situation calls for.
Participates in some recreational activities or hobbies.	Often participates in recreational activities and hobbies.	Participates in, as well as creates, variety of own recreational activities and hobbies.
Moderate problems most of time, or mild problems almost continuously.	Occasional moderate problems.	Occasional mild problems.
Almost equal in positive and negative attitude toward self.	Positive attitude toward self much of the time.	Positive attitude toward self most of the time.

Comments:

Developmentally Disabled PES Form 2: Goals

Screening _____
Initial _____
Reeval. No. _____
Closing _____

Client _____ CR TD DX UA OT
M/F/O—Sig. Other _____ CR TD DX UA OT
Therapist _____

Date _____
Case # _____

Name _____

INSTRUCTIONS—2
Please circle one in each column that describes best how you expect to be in _____ months.

Family Interaction	Occupation (School, Job or Homemaking)	Getting Along with Others	Feelings and Mood	Use of Free Time	Problems	Attitude toward Self
Often must have help with basic needs (for example, feeding, dressing, toilet).	Does not participate in planned program (such as Spec. Ed., Day Activities, or Sheltered Workshop) or work.	Always fighting or destructive; or always alone.	Almost always feels nervous, or depressed, or angry and bitter, or no emotions at all.	Almost no recreational activities or hobbies.	Severe problems most of the time.	Negative attitude toward self most of the time.
Occasionally needs some help with dressing, feeding, or toilet; able to help others when asked.	Is occasionally participating in planned program or work (up to 25% of the time).	Seldom able to get along with others without quarreling or being destructive; or is often alone.	Often feels nervous, or depressed, or angry and bitter, or hardly shows any emotion for weeks at a time.	Only occasional recreational activities, or repeats the same activity over and over again.	Severe problems some of the time or moderate problems continuously.	Negative attitude toward self much of the time.

Takes care of self and sometimes helps with home chores.	Often participates in planned program or work (between 25% and 50% of the time).	Sometimes quarreling, but seldom destructive; difficulties in making friends.	Frequently in a good mood but occasionally feels nervous, or depressed, or angry for days at a time.	Participates in some recreational activities or hobbies.	Moderate problems most of time, or mild problems almost continuously.	Almost equal in positive and negative attitude toward self.
Takes care of self and assumes regularly assigned responsibilities in the home.	Usually participates in planned program or work (between 50% and 75% of the time).	Gets along with others most of the time; has occasional friends.	Usually in a good mood, but occasionally feels nervous, or unhappy, or angry all day.	Often participates in recreational activities and hobbies.	Occasional moderate problems.	Positive attitude toward self much of the time.
Takes care of self and shares responsibilities and planning with others in the home.	Almost always participates in planned program or work (over 75% of the time).	Gets along with others most of the time; has regular friends.	In a good mood most of the time, and usually able to be as happy, or sad, or angry as the situation calls for.	Participates in, as well as creates, variety of own recreational activities and hobbies.	Occasional mild problems.	Positive attitude toward self most of the time.

Comments:

Bibliography

Albers, R.J. 1977. Patient satisfaction: Problems and prospects. *Psychiatric Outpatient Centers of America* 11:11–14.

Baron, F. 1953. An ego-strength scale which predicts response to psychotherapy. *Journal of Consulting Psychology* 17:327–333.

Bergin, A.E., and Suinn, R.M. 1975. Individual psychotherapy and behavior therapy. In M.R. Rosenzweig and L.W. Porter, eds., *Annual Review of Psychology*. Palo Alto: Annual Reviews.

Campbell, D.T., and Fiske, D.W. 1959. Convergent and discriminant validation by the multi-trait multi-method matrix. *Psychological Bulletin* 56:81–105.

Ciarlo, J.A., and Reihman, J. 1974. The Denver Community Mental Health Questionnaire. Unpublished manuscript. (Available from J.A. Ciarlo, Mental Health Systems Evaluation Project, 70 West Sixth Avenue, Denver, Colorado 80204.)

Cowen, E.L. 1978. Some problems in community program evaluation research. *Journal of Consulting and Clinical Psychology* 46:792–805.

Cronbach, L.J.; Gleser, G.C.; Nanda, H.; and Rajaratnam, N. 1972. *The Dependability of Behavioral Measurements: Theory of Generalizability for Scores and Profiles*. New York: Wiley.

Endicott, J.A., and Spitzer, R.L. 1972. What! Another rating scale? The psychiatric evaluation form. *Journal of Nervous and Mental Disease* 154:88–104.

Fenichel, O. 1945. *The Psychoanalytic Theory of Neurosis*. New York: Norton.

Freud, S. 1909. Analysis of a phobia in a five-year-old boy. In S. Freud, *Collected Papers*, Vol. 3. New York: Basic Books. 1959.

Freud, S. 1912. Recommendations for physicians on the psychoanalytic method of treatment. In S. Freud, *Collected Papers*, Vol. 2. New York: Basic Books, 1959.

Garfield, S.L. 1971. Research on client variables in psychotherapy. In A.E. Bergin and S.L. Garfield, eds. *Handbook of Psychotherapy and Behavior Change*. New York: Wiley.

Garfield, S.L.; Prager, R.A.; and Bergin, A.E. 1971. Evaluation of outcome in psychotherapy. *Journal of Consulting and Clinical Psychology* 37:301–313.

Gleser, G.C., and Ihilevich, D. 1969. An objective instrument for measuring defense mechanisms. *Journal of Consulting and Clinical Psychology* 33:51–60.

Gleser, G.C.; Seligman, R.; Winget, C.; and Rauh, J.L. 1977. Adolescents view their mental health. *Journal of Youth and Adolescence* 6:249–263.

Gleser, G.C.; Seligman, R.; Winget, C.; and Rauh, J.L. 1980. Parents view their adolescents' mental health. *Journal of Adolescent Health Care* 1:930–936.

Green, B.L.; Gleser, G.C.; Stone, W.N.; and Seifert, R.F. 1975. Relationship among diverse measures of psychotherapy outcome. *Journal of Consulting and Clinical Psychology* 43:689–699.

Jahoda, M. 1958. *Current Concepts of Positive Mental Health*. New York: Basic Books.

Katz, M.M., and Lyerly, S.B. 1963. Methods for measuring adjustment and social behavior in the community: Rationale, description, discriminative validity, and scale development. *Psychological Reports* 13:505–535.

Kiresuk, T.J., and Sherman, R.E. 1968. Goal attainment scaling: A general method for evaluating comprehensive community mental health programs. *Community Mental Health Journal* 4:443–453.

Offer, D., and Sabshin, M. 1966. *Normality: Theoretical and Clinical Concepts of Mental Health*. New York: Basic Books.

Perloff, R.; Perloff, E.; and Sussna, E. 1976. Program evaluation. In M.R. Rosenzweig and L.W. Porter, eds., *Annual Review of Psychology*. Palo Alto: Annual Reviews.

Rotter, J.B. 1966. Generalized expectancies for internal versus external control of reinforcement. *Psychological Monographs*, 80 (Whole No. 609).

Soddy, K., and Ahrenfeldt, R.H., eds. 1967. *Mental Health and Contemporary Thought*. London: Tavistock.

Strupp, H.H., and Hadley, S.W. 1977. A tripartite model of mental health and therapeutic outcomes with special reference to negative effects in psychotherapy. *American Psychologist* 32:187–196.

Taylor, J.A. 1953. A personality scale of manifest anxiety. *Journal of Abnormal and Social Psychology* 48:285–290.

Index of Names

Index of Subjects

About the Authors

Goldine C. Gleser received the Ph.D. in psychology from Washington University. She is currently professor emeritus of psychology in the Department of Psychiatry, University of Cincinnati College of Medicine. Her publications include books and articles on psychometric theory and applications, verbal behavior analysis, clinical evaluation, and disaster research.

David Ihilevich received the Ph.D. in clinical psychology from the University of Cincinnati. Since 1969 he has been the director of Shiawassee County Community Mental Health Center. His main research interests are in the area of defense mechanisms and evaluation of community mental-health services.